Vagus

Nerve

Healing

The Complete Guide on Vagus Nerve
Stimulating Exercises That Increase and
Activate Your Body's Natural Self-
Healing Power

Warren Hardy

TABLE OF CONTENTS

INTRODUCTION

Inflammation occurs as a natural and important function of the body's immune system and contributes to fighting infections. But when that system malfunctions, it can lead to continuing inflation; that, in turn, can lead to chronic illnesses, from Type 2 diabetes and arthritis to sepsis and atherosclerosis.

Managing that tension, easing that stress, reducing that inflammation may be brought under our control, in many cases, easily with certain maneuvers and exercises we'll be covering. These exercises, which include stretches, poses, muscular contractions and releases, and a range of managed breathing actions, work because they isolate the physical cause of the tension, the anxiety, the stress. The instigator is the vagus nerve, endowed by evolution to stimulate the fight or flight reactions that kept our ancestors safe when those real, existential threats were encountered. And while the vagus nerve gets our physical and emotional responses into high gear, it also can be stimulated to induce the calming effects that will bring us back down and into a state of stability and inner peace. The key is to strengthen the vagus nerve, achieving what is known as vagal tone.

The influences of the ubiquitous vagus nerve reach from the brainstem to our hearts and lungs, our digestive system, and to other essential organs, as well as controlling our ears, nose, throat and facial muscles. It can perform all of these functions, from a smile to a breath to a heartbeat, to a digestive action, because, like the other 11 cranial nerves, it's actually a double set of nerves. But unlike the others, the vagus nerve is the longest, most multitasked; no surprise that it has earned its reputation as the wanderer.

We'll begin our understanding of the vagus nerve with a look at our 12 cranial nerves and how they operate with the autonomic nervous system; a network that operates without our awareness and without our conscious help, to run our minds and bodies 24 hours a day without pause for rest or recuperation. This will lead to a look into the workings of the two nervous systems, the parasympathetic and the sympathetic, where physical and emotional responses—somatic and motor nerve functions—are generated and managed. These nervous systems react to evolutionary stimuli, pumping us up or cooling us down as required.

The most important motor functions deserve further understanding: the vagus nerve's effects on the oral cavity, the heartbeat, breathing, and digestion. We'll then move on to a newer discovery called the Polyvagal Theory, which postulates that certain physical actions, especially facial expressions, create what are called afferent influences on other parts of the body. This theory is still being tested, but there are encouraging indications of its validity.

Vagus nerve stimulation is important enough to cover in-depth, showing you certain movements, exercises, stretches and controlled breathing practices that can give you conscious control over your vagus nerve and how it influences both somatic and motor functions. The next discussion is dedicated to the electrical stimulation that medical professionals use to control heart rate and arrhythmia, and in treating gastroesophageal diseases, and to control the seizures of epilepsy. We'll then move on to the more experimental forms of vagus nerve stimulation, currently being tested for slowing the progression of Alzheimer's Disease and conditions within the Asperger's Spectrum, and, finally, we'll cover the impacts of vagus nerve injuries, including digestive gastroparesis, overreactions like vasovagal syncope and other results of overstimulation.

We'll conclude our voyage alongside the wandering vagus nerve with a recap of what you can do to more effectively manage your reactions and bring them under control as you sit, lie down, walk, participate in Yoga poses and stretches, and experience the immediate effects of managed breathing.

DISEASES ASSOCIATED WITH THE VAGUS NERVE AND HOW TO PREVENT THEM

Gastroparesis

Gastroparesis is a condition that influences the typical unconstrained development of the muscles (motility) in your stomach. Conventionally, solid strong compressions impel nourishment through your stomach related tract. Be that as it may, in the event that you have gastroparesis, your stomach's motility is backed off or doesn't work by any means, keeping it from discharging appropriately.

Certain prescriptions, for example, narcotic torment relievers, a few antidepressants, and hypertension and hypersensitivity drugs, can prompt moderate gastric exhausting and cause comparable side effects. For individuals who as of now have gastroparesis, these prescriptions may exacerbate their condition.

Gastroparesis can meddle with typical assimilation, cause sickness and retching, and cause issues with glucose levels and sustenance. The reason for gastroparesis is typically obscure. Once in a while it's an entanglement of diabetes, and a few people create gastroparesis after medical procedure. Despite the fact that there's no remedy for gastroparesis, changes to your eating regimen, alongside drug, can offer some help.

Side Effects

Signs and side effects of gastroparesis include:

- Vomiting
- Nausea
- Vomiting undigested nourishment eaten a couple of hours sooner
- Acid reflux
- Abdominal swelling
- Abdominal torment
- Changes in glucose levels
- Lack of craving
- Weight misfortune and unhealthiness

Numerous individuals with gastroparesis don't have any recognizable signs and side effects.

Causes

It's not in every case clear what prompts gastroparesis. Yet, much of the time, gastroparesis is accepted to be brought about by harm to a nerve that controls the stomach muscles (vagus nerve).

The vagus nerve deals with the intricate procedures in your stomach-related tract, incorporating flagging the muscles in your stomach to agreement and push nourishment into the small digestive tract. A harmed vagus nerve can't send flag typically to your stomach muscles. This may make nourishment stay in your stomach longer, instead of move regularly into your small digestive system to be processed.

The vagus nerve can be harmed by sicknesses, for example, diabetes, or by medical procedure to the stomach or small digestive system.

Hazard Factors

Components that can build your danger of gastroparesis:

- Diabetes
- Abdominal or esophageal medical procedure
- Infection, generally an infection
- Certain meds that moderate the pace of stomach discharging, for example, opiate torment meds
- Scleroderma (a connective tissue ailment)
- Nervous framework ailments, for example, Parkinson's ailment or various sclerosis
- Hypothyroidism (low thyroid)

Ladies are bound to create gastroparesis than men.

Difficulties

Gastroparesis can cause a few difficulties, for example,

- Severe lack of hydration. Continuous spewing can cause lack of hydration.
- Malnutrition. Poor hunger can mean you don't take in enough calories, or you might be not be able assimilate enough supplements because of regurgitating.

- Undigested nourishment that solidifies and stays in your stomach. Undigested nourishment in your stomach can solidify into a strong mass called a bezoar. Bezoars can cause queasiness and spewing and might be dangerous in the event that they keep nourishment from going into your small digestive system.
- Unpredictable glucose changes. In spite of the fact that gastroparesis doesn't cause diabetes, periodic changes in the rate and measure of nourishment going into the little entrails can cause inconsistent changes in glucose levels. These varieties in glucose exacerbate diabetes. Thus, poor control of glucose levels exacerbates gastroparesis.
- Decreased personal satisfaction. An intense erupt of side effects can make it hard to work and stay aware of different duties.

Seizure Disorders

In seizure issue, the cerebrum's electrical action is occasionally upset, bringing about some level of brief mind brokenness.

- Many individuals have uncommon sensations just before a seizure begins.
- Some seizures cause wild shaking and loss of awareness; however, more regularly, individuals essentially quit moving or become ignorant of what's going on.
- Doctors suspect the conclusion dependent on indications, yet imaging of the mind, blood tests, and electroencephalography (to record the cerebrum's electrical action) are generally expected to recognize the reason.

- If required, medications can, for the most part, help avert seizures.

Ordinary mind capacity requires a deliberate, composed, facilitated release of electrical driving forces. Electrical motivations empower the mind to speak with the spinal line, nerves, and muscles just as inside itself. Seizures may result when the cerebrum's electrical action is disturbed.

About 2% of grown-ups have a seizure eventually during their life. 66% of these individuals never have another. Seizure issue usually start in early adolescence or in late adulthood.

Kinds of Seizures

Seizures might be depicted as pursues:

- Epileptic: These seizures have no clear trigger (that is, they are ridiculous), and they happen at least multiple times. One seizure isn't viewed as epilepsy. Epileptic seizures are known as a seizure issue or epilepsy. What causes epileptic seizures is regularly obscure (called idiopathic epilepsy). Be that as it may, they might be brought about by different cerebrum issue, for example, auxiliary anomalies, strokes, or tumors. In such cases, they are called symptomatic epilepsy. Symptomatic epilepsy is most regular among infants and more seasoned individuals.
- Non-epileptic: These seizures are activated (incited) by a reversible issue or a condition that disturbs the cerebrum, for example, a contamination, a stroke, head damage, or a

response to a medication. In youngsters, a fever can trigger a non-epileptic seizure (called a febrile seizure).

Causes

The causes usually depend on when seizures start:

- Before age 2: High fevers or transitory metabolic variations from the norm, for example, unusual blood levels of sugar (glucose), calcium, magnesium, nutrient B6, or sodium, can trigger at least one seizures. Seizures don't happen once the fever or variation from the norm settle. On the off chance that the seizures repeat without such triggers, the reason is probably going to be damage during birth, a birth imperfection, or an inherited metabolic variation from the norm or mind issue.
- 2 to 14 years: Often, the reason is obscure.
- Adults: Head damage, stroke, or tumor may harm the mind, causing a seizure. Liquor withdrawal (brought about by abruptly halting drinking) is a typical reason for seizures.
- Older grown-ups: The reason might be a cerebrum tumor or stroke.

Seizures with no recognizable reason are called idiopathic.

Conditions that aggravate the cerebrum, for example, wounds, certain medications, lack of sleep, contaminations, fever—or that deny the mind of oxygen or fuel, for example, unusual heart rhythms, a low degree of oxygen in the blood, or an extremely low degree of sugar in the blood (hypoglycemia)— can trigger a solitary seizure whether an individual has a seizure issue or not. A seizure that comes from such an upgrade is known as an incited seizure (and in this manner is a non-epileptic seizure).

Individuals with a seizure issue are bound to have a seizure when the following happen:

- They are under abundance physical or passionate pressure.
- They are inebriated or denied of rest.
- They have all of a sudden quit drinking or using tranquilizers.

Maintaining a strategic distance from these conditions can help avert seizures.

Seldom, seizures are activated by tedious sounds, blazing lights, computer games, or in any event, contacting certain pieces of the body. In such cases, the turmoil is called reflex epilepsy.

Manifestations

A quality (bizarre sensations) depicts how an individual feels before a seizure starts, or it might be a piece of a central mindful seizure that is simply beginning. An air may incorporate any of he following:

- Abnormal scents or tastes
- Butterflies in the stomach

- Feeling as though something has been experienced before despite the fact that it has not (called this feels familiar) or the contrary inclination—something appears to be new despite the fact that it is commonplace here and there (called jamais vu)
- An extraordinary inclination that a seizure is going to start.
- Practically all seizures are moderately concise, enduring from a couple of moments to a couple of minutes. Most seizures last 1 to 2 minutes.

Every so often, seizures repeat over and again, as happens in status epilepticus.

The vast majority who have a seizure issue look and act regularly between seizures.

Side effects of seizures differ contingent upon which zone of the mind is influenced by the strange electrical release, as in the following:

- An strongly lovely or upsetting taste if the piece of the cerebrum called the insula is influenced
- Visual mind flights (seeing unformed pictures) if the occipital flap is influenced
- Inability to talk if the territory that controls discourse (situated in the frontal flap) is influenced
- A seizure (snapping and fits of muscles all through the body) if huge territories on the two sides of the mind are influenced
- Seizures might be delegated

- Motor: Involving anomalous muscle compressions, (for example, jolting of an appendage or seizures)
- Non-motor: Not including anomalous muscle compressions

Other potential indications incorporate deadness or shivering in a particular body part, brief scenes of lethargy, loss of awareness, and disarray. Individuals may upchuck on the off chance that they lose awareness. Individuals may lose control of their muscles, bladder, or guts. A few people keep quiet.

Side effects additionally differ contingent upon whether the seizure is:

- Focal-beginning (the seizure starts in a single side of the mind)
- Generalized-beginning (the seizure starts in the two sides of the mind)

There are a few sorts of central and summed-up seizures. The vast majority have just one sort of seizure. Others have at least two sorts.

A few kinds of seizures might be central or summed up:

- Atonic (including loss of muscle tone)
- Clonic (including cadenced snapping of muscles)
- Tonic (including hardening of muscles)
- Myoclonic (including abrupt, lightning-like snapping of muscles)
- Epileptic (juvenile) fits and febrile seizures, which happen in kids

Central Beginning Seizures

In central beginning seizures, the seizures start in one side of the cerebrum. These seizures are ordered dependent on whether the individual knows during the seizure:

- Awareness is kept up (called central mindful seizures).
- Awareness is disabled (called central debilitated mindfulness seizures).

Mindfulness alludes to learning of self and condition. On the off chance that mindfulness is weakened during any piece of the seizure, the seizure is viewed as a central hindered mindfulness seizure. Specialists decide if individuals stayed mindful during a seizure by asking them or, if a seizure is happening, checking whether they react when addressed.

In central mindful seizures, strange electrical releases start in a little zone of the cerebrum and stay limited to that zone. Since just a little zone of the mind is influenced, side effects are identified with the capacity constrained by that territory. For instance, if the little region of the cerebrum that controls the correct arm's developments (in the left frontal projection) is influenced, the correct arm may automatically be lifted up and snap, and the head may move in the direction of the lifted arm. Individuals are totally cognizant and mindful of the environment. A central mindful seizure may advance to a central debilitated mindfulness seizure.

Jacksonian seizures are a kind of central mindful seizures. Side effects start in one hand or foot, and at that point climb the appendage as the electrical action spreads in the cerebrum. Individuals are totally mindful of what is happening during the seizure.

Other central mindful seizures influence the face, and at that point spread to an arm or now and again a leg.

In central impeded mindfulness seizures, unusual electrical releases start in a little territory of the worldly flap or frontal projection and immediately spread to other close-by zones. The seizures start with an air, which keeps going 1 to 2 minutes. During the atmosphere, individuals begin to put some distance between the environment.

During the seizure, mindfulness winds up disabled; however, individuals don't end up oblivious. Individuals may do the following:

- Stare
- Chew or smack the lips automatically
- Move the hands, arms, and legs in abnormal, purposeless ways
- Utter useless sounds
- Not comprehend what other individuals are stating
- Resist help

A few people can chat; however, their discussion needs immediacy, and the substance is, to some degree, scanty. They might be confounded and muddled. This state may keep going for a few minutes. Every so often, individuals lash out in the event that they are limited.

A few people at that point recuperate completely. In others, the strange electrical release spreads to contiguous territories and to the opposite side of the mind, bringing about a summed-up seizure. Summed-up seizures that result from central seizures are called central to two-sided seizures. That is, they start in one side of the mind and spread to the two sides.

Epilepsia partialis continua is uncommon. Central seizures happen at regular intervals or minutes for quite a long time to years one after another. They commonly influence an arm, a hand, or one side of the face. These seizures result from:

- In grown-ups: Localized cerebrum harm, (for example, scarring because of a stroke)
- In youngsters: Inflammation of the mind (as happens in encephalitis and measles)

Summed-Up Beginning Seizures

In summed-up beginning seizures, the seizure starts in the two sides of the cerebrum. Most summed-up beginning seizures disable mindfulness. They frequently cause loss of awareness and anomalous developments, normally right away. Loss of cognizance might be brief or keep going quite a while.

Summed-up beginning seizures incorporate the following sorts:

- Tonic-clonic seizures (some time ago, called fabulous mal seizures)

- Clonic seizures
- Tonic seizures
- Atonic seizures
- Myoclonic seizures, including adolescent myoclonic epilepsy
- Epileptic (juvenile) fits
- Absence seizures

Most kinds of summed-up seizures, (for example, tonic-clonic seizures) include strange muscle withdrawals. Those that don't are called nonattendance seizures.

In summed-up tonic-clonic seizures, muscles contract (the tonic part), and at that point quickly shift back and forth among contracting and unwinding (the clonic part). These seizures might be:

- Generalized (beginning in the two sides of the mind)
- Focal to two-sided (beginning in one side of the mind and spreading to the two sides)

In the two sorts, awareness is incidentally lost and a seizure happens when the unusual releases spread to the two sides of the mind.

Summed-up beginning seizures start with irregular releases in a profound, focal piece of the mind and spread all the while to the two sides of the cerebrum. There is no emanation. The seizure regularly starts with a clamor. Individuals at that point become uninformed or lose awareness.

During summed-up beginning seizures, individuals may do the following:

- Have serious muscle fits and yanking all through the body
- Fall down
- Clench their teeth
- Bite their tongue (regularly happens)
- Drool or foam at the mouth
- Lose control of the bladder and additionally entrails

The seizures generally last 1 to 2 minutes. A short time later, a few people, who have a cerebral pain, are incidentally confounded and feel very drained. These indications may last from minutes to hours. A great many people don't recollect what occurred during the seizure.

Central to-reciprocal tonic-clonic (fabulous mal) seizures for the most part start with an unusual electrical release in a little zone of one side of the cerebrum, bringing about a central mindful or central weakened mindfulness seizure. The release at that point rapidly spreads to the two sides of the mind, making the whole cerebrum glitch. Indications are like those of summed-up beginning seizures.

Atonic seizures happen fundamentally in youngsters. They are described by a brief, however complete loss of muscle tone and awareness. They cause kids to tumble to the ground, some of the time bringing about damage.

In clonic seizures, the appendages on the two sides of the body and frequently head, neck, face, and trunk snap musically all through the seizure. Clonic seizures more often than not happen in newborn children. They are considerably less basic than tonic-clonic seizures.

Tonic seizures happen regularly during rest, typically in kids. Muscle tone increments unexpectedly or step by step, making muscles harden. The appendages and neck are regularly influenced. Tonic seizures commonly last just 10 to 15 seconds, however can cause individuals, if remaining, to tumble to the ground. The vast majority don't lose awareness. On the off chance that seizures last more, muscles may twitch a couple of times as the seizure closes.

Atypical nonattendance seizures, atonic seizures, and tonic seizures typically happen as a major aspect of a serious type of epilepsy called Lennox-Gastaut disorder, which starts before kids are 4 years of age.

Myoclonic seizures are described by one or a few appendages or the storage compartment. The seizures are brief and don't cause loss of cognizance; however, they may happen drearily and may advance to a tonic-clonic seizure with loss of awareness.

Adolescent myoclonic epilepsy commonly starts during immaturity. Regularly, seizures start with brisk rascals of the two arms. About 90% of these seizures are trailed by tonic-clonic seizures. A few people additionally have nonattendance seizures. The seizures frequently happen when individuals stir toward the beginning of the day, particularly on the off chance that they are restless. Drinking liquor additionally makes these seizures more probable.

Nonappearance seizures don't include irregular muscle compression. They might be delegated

- Typical (petit mal)
- Atypical

Common nonattendance seizures for the most part start in adolescence, more often than not between the ages of 5 and 15 years, and don't proceed into adulthood. In any case, grown-ups once in a while have commonplace nonappearance seizures. Dissimilar to tonic-clonic seizures, nonattendance seizures don't cause spasms or other sensational side effects. Individuals don't tumble down, break down, or move jerkily. Rather, they have scenes of gazing with rippling eyelids and here and there jerking facial muscles. They ordinarily lose cognizance, winding up totally unconscious of their environment. These scenes last 10 to 30 seconds. Individuals unexpectedly stop what they are doing and continue it similarly as suddenly. They experience no eventual outcomes and don't have a clue that a seizure has happened. Without treatment, numerous individuals have a few seizures every day. Seizures regularly happen when individuals are sitting discreetly. Seizures seldom happen during activity. Hyperventilation can trigger a seizure.

Atypical nonappearance seizures differ from commonplace nonattendance seizures in the following ways:

- They are less normal.
- They last more.
- Jerking and different developments are progressively articulated.
- People are increasingly mindful of their environment.

A great many people with atypical nonappearance seizures have neurologic variations from the norm or formative postponements. Atypical nonattendance seizures as a rule proceed into adulthood.

Status epilepticus

Convulsive status epilepticus is the most genuine seizure issue and is viewed as a health-related crisis in light of the fact that the seizure doesn't stop. Electrical releases happen all through the cerebrum, causing a summed-up tonic-clonic seizure.

Convulsive status epilepticus is analyzed when either of the following happens:

- A seizure lasts over 5 minutes
- People don't totally recapture awareness between at least two seizures

Individuals have seizures with exceptional muscle withdrawals and frequently can't inhale enough. Body temperature increments. Without quick treatment, the heart and cerebrum can move toward becoming overburdened and for all time harmed, now and again bringing about death.

Summed-up convulsive status epilepticus has numerous causes, including harming the head and unexpectedly halting an anti-seizure tranquilize.

Non-convulsive status epilepticus, another kind of status epilepticus, doesn't cause spasms. The seizures happen for 10 minutes or more. During the seizure, mental procedures (counting mindfulness) and additionally conduct are influenced. Individuals may seem befuddled or scattered. They might not be able to talk and may carry on nonsensically. Having non-convulsive status epilepticus expands the danger of creating convulsive status epilepticus. This kind of seizure requires brief conclusion and treatment.

Indications After a Seizure

At the point when a seizure stops, individuals may have a cerebral pain, sore muscles, bizarre sensations, perplexity, and significant weariness. These eventual outcomes are known as the post-ictal state. In certain individuals, one side of the body is feeble after a seizure, and the shortcoming keeps going longer than the seizure (a confusion called Todd loss of motion).

A great many people don't recall what occurred during the seizure (a condition called post-ictal amnesia).

Difficulties

Seizures may have genuine outcomes. Serious, fast muscle compressions can cause wounds, including broken bones. Unexpected loss of cognizance can cause genuine damage because of falls and mishaps. Individuals may have various seizures without bringing about genuine mind harm. In any case, seizures that repeat and cause spasms may inevitably impede insight.

In the event that seizures are not well-controlled, individuals might be not able get a driver's permit. They may experience issues keeping a vocation or getting protection. They might be socially vilified. Subsequently, their personal satisfaction might be generously decreased.

In the event that seizures are not totally controlled, individuals are a few times bound to pass on than the individuals who don't have seizures.

A couple of individuals kick the bucket all of a sudden for no clear reason—an entanglement called abrupt surprising passing in epilepsy. This issue happens around evening time or during rest. Hazard is most noteworthy for individuals who have visit seizures, particularly summed-up tonic-clonic seizures.

Analysis

- A specialist's assessment
- If the individual has never had a seizure, blood and different tests, imaging of the mind, and generally electroencephalography
- If a seizure issue has just been analyzed, typically blood tests to quantify levels of antiseizure drugs

Specialists analyze a seizure issue when individuals have at any rate two unjustifiable seizures that happen at various occasions. The finding depends on indications and the perceptions of observers. Manifestations that recommend a seizure incorporate loss of awareness, muscle fits that shake the body, loss of bladder control, abrupt disarray, and powerlessness to focus. In any case, seizures cause such indications substantially less regularly than the vast majority think. A short loss of cognizance is bound to swoon (syncope) than a seizure.

Individuals are typically assessed in a crisis division. On the off chance that a seizure issue has just been analyzed and individuals have totally recuperated, they might be assessed in a specialist's office.

HOW DOES SPD AFFECT DAILY LIFE?

T hough it is a true neurological dysfunction in which the brain does not respond to outside stimuli in an appropriate manner, SPD is not recognized as a medical diagnosis. Many times, a parent will need to research their child's "abnormalities" on their own and request a referral to an Occupational Therapist for assessment. Unless the OT can also find a clinical developmental delay that coincides with the SPD, their therapy services aren't covered by insurance because it's not a "medical diagnosis."

For families that choose to use an OT, therapy doesn't "cure" SPD. Treatment aims to heighten dulled senses or desensitize the overstimulated. Much of the success in SPD therapy comes from continuing the exercises at home on a long-term basis.

While some forms of sensory problems are evident, such as in kids with ADHD, Asperger's, or Autism, many children suffer from mild, hidden forms of an SPD. Many parents don't know there is a sensory problem, and they just know they have a "difficult" child. Some of these sensory issues can manifest as:

- Inconsistent potty training despite appropriate age
- Difficulty dressing or feeding themselves
- Extreme food aversions to taste, smell, and textures; Limited intake of food/nutrients
- Difficulty in fine motor skills like handwriting

- Difficulty in gross motor skills - very clumsy, poor body control/coordination
- Restlessness, fidgety, easily distracted
- Extremely sensitive to clothing and shoes - Fabric textures, tags, buttons, zippers, seams, etc.
- Extreme dislike (or joy) over teeth brushing, hair brushing, trips to the dentist, etc.

Many times, these children hold labels such as stubborn, defiant, and difficult. They appear overdramatic about little things. Teachers find them disruptive and frustrating to have in the classroom.

Even after a parent realizes that their child has a sensory problem and seeks treatment, life with the child will never be "normal." Through therapy, some kids can learn to tolerate certain sensations and stimuli, but they will always be different.

Living with an SPD is a life-long process of learning what senses get triggered and how to cope or respond. It is difficult to send your picky eater to a friend's house and explain to the mother why they don't like most foods. It is hard for others to purchase clothing or shoes, as the child needs specific fabrics or button placements or no seams. Your child may hold it together all day at school, but come home and meltdown because their senses are on overload.

Life with SPD is a constant battle for "normal" while knowing that you never will be. It is learning triggers and coping mechanisms so they can fit in with their peers. It is constant battles over what to eat for dinner or what to wear to school. It is frequent bumps and bruises and boxes of band-aids. It is fights and tears over the need to brush teeth or hair.

For many kids with special needs, their differences are apparent. For others, special needs are hidden and poorly understood. Kids with SPD - the ones who seem dramatic, defiant, stubborn, or inattentive - need patience, understanding, and tools to help them cope.

Psychopathologies

Psychopathology means the science of psychological disorders. On the other hand, it can be defined as the study of the nature of how abnormal behavior, thoughts, and feelings do develop. Some researchers term the survey to be ambiguous since it is hard to get the facts, but it is fun studying about it. The researchers develop efforts to entirely understand the biological, genetic, psychological, and social causes. The study of nosology involved can help improve some treatment outcomes of the diseases that come up during the development stages.

Diagnostic Systems of Psychopathology

All the medical professionals engaged in the research, analysis and treatment of psychopathology use the best diagnostic systems. With the networks, they can get reasonable conclusions, and get the most effective treatment for psychological disorders.

Distinguishing Psychopathology Vs. Normal Behavior

There are ways in which psychologists and the psychiatrists can decide to which extent normal behavior enters the psychopathology disorders territory. The disorders do touch four main areas that include the deviance, distress, danger, and pathology states.

Whenever you are determining whether a behavior is quite normal or not, one can consider if the responses do violate the standard expected social norms also, if it makes people feel a bit anxious or somewhat threatened. Most psychopaths do display antisocial behaviors. The behaviors do make people around the affected person feel uncomfortable.

However, the above is just a narrow definition. One can think of prostitutes and the criminals they do violate the social norms, but that does not mean they are abnormal. Also, social models vary from culture to culture. In some cultures, homosexuality is acceptable, whereas, in others, it is illegal.

For example, one can be experiencing some symptoms of depression, and you visit the psychiatrist. The doctor will most likely assess you according to the list of symptoms of the psychological disorders or abnormal behaviors below:

- Deviance, which refers to the person's thoughts, actions, or thoughts, which are not acceptable in society or directly in one's culture. In most cases where one is depressed, there is a tendency to feel guilty and worthless, which is not so familiar to other people.

- The second one is distress, where the affected person always has negative feelings towards themselves or to other people who are around them. When depressed, one feels exceptionally distressed, sad, and more so feels so guilty.
- Third, is when one feels body dysfunctional, it refers to the inability to be able to attend to your daily functions so well. For example, going to work and achieving the set goals. When depressed, you will not be able to get out of bed and do your daily activities. In case you decide to do them, they will take a much longer time than you do.
- Fourth, is a danger, which means a violent behavior towards people or yourself. When depressed, one can even have thoughts and feelings to harm yourself by committing suicide.

How Does It Help In Treating Psychopathologies?

The theory is used to solve a quite a list of psychiatric conditions. It spans the spectra used in internalizing and externalizing. It provides unique and clear insights into the primary role of the emotional deregulation in psychology and the notable development of some observable patterns. The patterns are from the autonomic nervous system. The models function in the clinical syndromes.

The Polyvagal Theory does provide a platform, which is theoretical for people in the clinical industry, to comprehend the interactions of the internal HPA axis that are functional. Also, they can appreciate the vasopressin of the autonomic nervous system. The neuropeptides of oxytocin are also understood.

The adrenal gland has structures that function well in exhibiting the phylogenic changes. However, the cortex in the adrenal is generally considered as the special endocrine organ. The substantial part of this axis is known as HPA. It was traditionally studied. Besides, researchers discussed it independently from the autonomic nervous system and the adrenal medulla. The cortex has a mesodermal origin, which is very different from the ectodermal. The ectodermal is home to the medulla.

There is corticoid that is secreted by the ductless glands. The secreted corticoid is used to reduce stress. All vertebrates that are alive do secrete the corticosteroids and catecholamine. It is essential always to note that the structures that do produce the secretions do follow the trend that is phylogenetic and mostly results in two or three anatomical alterations.

The medulla can receive a significant quantity of the corticosteroids mainly through the adrenaline vascular system. The hormones in there do activate the enzyme system for the work to convert norepinephrine to epinephrine. The effect ends up supporting the sympathetic adrenal medulla functions. The functions are as well associated with the increased metabolic activity and its metabolization also. It is a fact that epinephrine has a significant impact on blood glucose elevation. The glucose in blood concurrently influences the adrenal steroids.

On the other hand, hydrocortone does directly enhance the mobilization by bringing changes through gluconeogenesis in the liver. Through the process, the suckle changes to aldohexose. The process does contribute to the demands of metabolism through the increase in glucose available. Also, the reduction in oxygen debts since the lactate will be accumulated.

The vagal activity is generally implicated in the functions of the adrenal cortex. In a similar case, the psychological stressors can reduce the tone of the cardiac vagal, increasing the cortisol plasma levels. There is an increase in the sympathetic activations and the circulation of the catecholamine. In The Polyvagal Theory, there is the organic process where cortisol secretions are related to the maintenance of the mobilizations. An example of the mobilization process is the conversion of norepinephrine to epinephrine. The process is done during a fight.

Through research, it is determined that all, crawling and walking, vertebrates possess the peptides that are similar in cellular structure with the vasopressin and the oxytocin. On the other hand, it is known that only mammals have receptors that are very specific for both the peptides. The vasopressin and oxytocin are primarily synthesized. The process takes place in the supraoptic, and the periventricular nuclei of the earlier discussed hypothalamus. They are later released to the organs via the parvocellular neurons. It is done systematically through the magnocellular neurons.

There are different systemic and central effects of the neuropeptides involved. There is the first release of the hormone oxytocin that regulates the dorsal motor nucleus outputs. The outputs are well maintained within the levels that are optimal to help in supporting the homeostasis process. Also, it provides an excellent anti-stress state. Also, the endocrine got the peripheral unharness that expounds the functions related to ejections, uterine contractions as well as sperm ejaculations. The central releasing of the vasopressin does appear to modulate the afferent feedbacks from the shifted setpoint and the viscera. It is, however, independent of the vagal reflexes sensitivities that include the baroreceptor reflex.

Also, there is raising the set point in the baroreceptors. Doctors accomplish these by increasing cardiac output. There is potential in fight-flight behaviors that do allow the sympathetic excitation of the heart. The vagal reflexes that are homeostatic do not oppose the excitation. The intermediate levels of vasopressin are as well considered to have a relation with the tender processes. Since the peripheral processes do influence the vasopressin and the oxytocin functions through the DVC sensory component, it is a primary process, and the peripheral effects of the peptides are not so apparent. They may differ as to the function of acute as compared to chronic exposure. To support the above speculation, in humans, it is well known that the peripheral vasopressin is the one that is related to nausea, not oxytocin.

The hormone oxytocin is also part of the response, which is posh and is associated with a high setting. In the past, the theory has coherently been in use in an extensive range of clinical observations. The approach has as well provided precise and in-depth insights concerning the role of emotions. Deregulation in psychopathology and progressive development of aberrant patterns is utilized in the autonomic nervous system.

A researcher in the past hypothesized the relations involved in the biological risks to acquire a syndrome. It is important to note that impulsivity, which is somehow inherited, may render the ADHD children at a high risk of developing the CD in the future. It also happens in families that have coercive environments, in cases where emotional liability is normally reinforced in a repeated manner. In the past system, functioning has always been considered unrelated in the many clinical syndromes.

The theory has generated a very good host for all the detailed insights that researchers may never have pursued even now. When children have strong emotions when they are socializing, chances are there will be reduced risk of kids with ADHD developing CD. It has been researched that ADHD automatically leads to CD when the bringing up of the children is accompanied by ultimate coercive parenting.

The autonomic and the emotional liability in children are shaped through the repeated exposure of the negative effects where CD development is quite encouraged. It is a simple implication that the autonomic markers through the emotional lability that is inclusive of the RSA are responsive to the psychological issues. The psychological interventions do target the coercive interaction patterns that are even able to promote social competence.

Through the context of the theory, kids who are aggressive with the ODD or CD do appear to be mostly in the double jeopardy, which is not a pleasing state. In the first place, they tend to exhibit under arousal, which is sympathetic at a very early age. Also, they do experience the sympathetic insensitivity, which marks a very general tendency of disinhibitory. The disinhibition process is accompanied by some deficiencies that lead to greater emotional lability. The children are put at risk of having psychopathological conditions. The conditions do cover the whole externalizing spectrum. However, there is a theory that chronic activities in the central dopamine are connected to various identifiable disinhibitory conditions. The conditions include; ADHD, excessive drinking problems, and related substance abuse, among others.

As in The Polyvagal Theory, the response strategies are mediated in the SNS. They do predominate when the functions of the emotions regulatory as served by the PNS fails. The features are served via the smartest vagus. The results are likely to represent some failures in the development of the affected people. The individuals do not normally acquire self-regulatory body functions. The Polyvagal Theory does suggest that the difficulties observed in the areas. They are marked by the vagal tones that are attenuated. The failure of the smart vagus processes can inhibit behaviors that are proponent, whereas the attentional allocation is quite adaptive. The modulation of the emotions may make kids with CD have no viable response. Thus, they will not be able to get mechanisms that can inhibit impulsive and labile behaviors.

The Polyvagal Theory predicts that the vagal deficiencies are mostly observed in children as well as adolescents that are aggressive. Also, there is a phylogenic approach. It does emphasize on the avoidance, and the defense behaviors do have the vagal components that are manifested through DVC. An example is when one experiences physiological shutdown as mediated by DVC, there is a likelihood the affected person will support avoidance behaviors such as feigning of death.

The theory does force people to have a different perspective on the interpretation of social behaviors. It emphasizes merely how social practices are limited only to the psychological states of people. It states that the immobilization and mobilization behaviors may be adaptive to an individual who is frightened.

In conclusion, the theory does provide a platform that is theoretical on how to interpret the social behaviors, especially in neurophysiological context.

- Learn to manage your emotions

Behaviors are the result of feelings, and feelings are the result of thoughts. Thus, if you can begin to change the way you think, you can inevitably change your behavior. This is the basic principle behind cognitive-behavioral therapy. Your cognitive state and your behavior are connected. Undesired behaviors, such as anxiety or depression, can then be lessened, if not entirely eradicated, simply by discovering the thought processes that began the downward spiral into your depressed state. Here are just a few of the many benefits of cognitive-behavioral therapy.

- Identifies the cause of your behavior

Behaving in a way that is unfavorable to you without knowing why or how to stop yourself is frustrating. Let's say, hypothetically, that you have an irrational fear of getting behind the wheel of a car. It interferes with your daily life, but you can't seem to fix this behavior. Your inability to change may be irritating, and you may struggle to find solutions, but unless you know the root cause of your problem, it will be difficult to make progress. Cognitive-behavioral therapy digs deep to uncover the origin of the undesired behavior. Perhaps the reason for your fear of driving directly relates to an accident you were involved in several years ago that left you traumatized. Your therapist can work with you to help you properly process that event in a way that will set you free from its long-term effects. This method can also be used for any other fear as well as addictions.

- Sets you free from your thoughts

Whether you're suffering from a condition as severe as depression, or merely being controlled by a minor bad habit, it is possible to be set free from your thoughts. How incredible would it be to recognize negative thoughts as they enter your mind and choose not to let them affect your mood? This doesn't mean you can control what you think, but you can absolutely control your response to those thoughts with a bit of hard work and practice.

- Creates happiness

You're a wonderful human being with gifts and talents to share with the world. You were created to live a full and happy life. Your mind should never have the power to prevent you from enjoying yourself and those around you. By being set free from whatever holds you back (i.e., anxiety, addictions, depression) through the use of therapy, you can begin to see the real you.

Understanding VNS Treatment

The cause of VNS is straightforward. It takes a stab at the vagus nerve, which is the longest cranial nerve in the human body going from the neck to the thorax and the intestines. This nerve assumes an urgent role in observing key capacities in the human body. In the event that there are varieties, for example, increased breathing, the vagus nerve transfers messages to the brain with respect to how to react. During

VNS treatment, the surgeon embeds a little device like a pacemaker beneath the neck which enacts the nerve.

Distrust with respect to the benefits of the treatment has stayed among the restorative clique, however its capacity as a bogus treatment has been opposed by therapist Prof. Hamish McAllister-Williams from Newcastle University. In spite of the fact that he concedes that very little is known about its viability in instances of serious despondency that stay static to conventional medications, he is certain that the effect of VNS isn't comparable to a bogus treatment. Bogus treatment is promptly actuated and closes rapidly, while VNS takes a half year before its effect can be felt.

In a recent report on depressed patients who were impervious to treatment, it was seen that the people furnished subordinate VNS alongside routine treatment for depression, the reaction rates were higher than when one just relied upon treatment as usual (TAU). Another study by therapist Scott Aaronson additionally uncovered that VNS when utilized with TAU would provide better long-term results than if there was an occurrence of just TAU.

Remarking on the investigation result, Aaronson stated, "The averageness of the gadget is tremendous. The principle symptom is dryness in light of the fact that the intermittent laryngeal nerve [that supplies the voice box] falls off the vagus nerve." He proposed that the reactions could be constrained by incidentally turning off the gadget by holding a magnet over it.

Aside from dryness in the voice, the treatment additionally causes successive coughing, breathing difficulties and changes in heart tone. It might likewise bring about one's death or psychosis upon becoming disturbed. Hence, it is important to exercise caution before prescribing bioelectric treatments for depression.

Elective medications for depression

There are numerous innovative treatments for combatting depression. Their utilization with standard medications is incredibly compelling for keeping the condition under control. Three such treatments that connect with one's concerns effectively while keeping negative thoughts under control are as below:

Workmanship treatment: One can participate in creative expressions even without having any related knowledge in dance or acting. These exercises open the body and brain to an alternate encounter and assist one with interfacing with him/herself. They help discharge all pessimism and lift confidence in this way lessening side effects of enduring trouble and low state of brain, and characteristics of despair.

Mindfulness treatment: Both Mindfulness-based stress reduction (MBSR) and Mindfulness-based cognitive therapy (MBCT) advance passionate success and stirs inspiration. Such treatments center around being in the present without agonizing over the past or future. They urge an individual to be responsive to one's senses and increase better understanding and control of their concerns and habits.

Eco treatment: As the name suggests, eco treatment encourages one to associate with nature. Regardless of whether it is through walks in nature or gardening, it depends on the capability of the nature to help you recuperate, ease and calm.

Try not to give despair a chance to damage your life

The World Health Organization (WHO) reports that depression is the main source of incapacity overall influencing a greater number of ladies than men. Be that as it may, with appropriate drugs and treatment, one can have a quality existence. It is essential to look for advice from a verified emotional wellness professional who can analyze the condition in time and propose suitable treatment.

Do You Know Where and What Your Vagus Is?

The meaning of vagus: vagus (Latin, vagus = meandering) cranial nerve X (CN X) a blended nerve that leaves the head and neck to innervate gastrointestinal tract (pharynx, throat, stomach) respiratory tract (larynx, lungs), cardiovascular (heart) and stomach viscera. This blended nerve has tactile, engine and autonomic elements of viscera (organs, digestion, pulse).

Indeed, you have one of these as we as a whole do, it is a long meandering nerve and it is the essential nerve interfacing the brain alongside each organ of the body. It regulates your pulse, your processing system, disposal and essentially all automated elements of your body. They additionally share the investigation of how the condition of your sensory system and your resistant system add to wellbeing and lifespan.

The vagus is straightforwardly connected with our development, it screens our sensory system and insusceptible system which legitimately adds to our wellbeing and lifespan. So as we age the greatest issues include inflammatory conditions in our bodies, and that is related straightforwardly with stress, living in the fast-track and ill-advised eating routines. So here we have one more zone of our bodies that we can keep stable and energetic to draw out our maturation process and indeed, keeping it sound is the reduction of stress and an absolute solid way of life.

What would we be able to do to calm the vagus and keep from untimely aging and to carry on with a long and upbeat life? It truly is basic, one is reflection, Chi-gong, guided perception and yoga, they all are fun, and are additionally extremely simple to do and just takes a brief period from your day.

Thought for the Afternoon: "We are starting to understand wellbeing not as the absence of illness, but instead as the procedure by which people keep up their feeling of lucidness (for example sense that life is understandable, reasonable, and significant) and capacity to work despite changes in themselves and their relationships with their condition.

The Polyvagal Hierarchy - Rules of Engagement

Ever wonder how the omnipresence of messaging will influence our development?

Neurophysiologist Stephen Porges, teacher of psychiatry at the University of North Carolina, focuses on the fact that physiological connectedness is an organic objective. He demonstrates this by referencing his polyvagal hypothesis, which depicts the capacity of the tenth cranial nerve, the vagus.

The vagus is a segment of the autonomic sensory system (ANS) which is the system that keeps imperative organs like the heart and lungs working. The ANS separates into the sympathetic and parasympathetic systems which spend and recharge physiological assets.

Porges recommends we focus on the zone around the eyes when conversing with somebody since "physiology decides brain research." If we have a sense of security when seeing benevolence in somebody's face, our vagus nerve acts as a "brake" on the pulse which, without the high vagal tone, would speed crazily. The vagus "represses" different practices, such as talking, which energizes tuning in.

The vagus nerve emerges from two separate cores in the brainstem which suits more established and more up to date branches. The unmyelinated more established branch slips down the back spine and innervates organs underneath the stomach. This "vegetative" vagus is basic to all vertebrates - including reptiles who stop when in danger.

The more modern myelinated vagal branch slides down the front spine and actuates organs over the stomach. This "savvy" vagus is shared by all well evolved creatures. Since well evolved creatures are subject to other warm blooded animals to survive, this vagus supports social commitment.

The seventh cranial nerve controls the face muscles and emerges from a similar core on the brainstem as the keen vagus. The facial nerve enacts the muscles around the eye, including the orbicularis oculi, which registers feeling. Prompts we read all over track again into the vagus and influence our physiology.

The fight or flight reaction is a part of the more modern vagus and emerges when we don't see a caring face, however a level face; or we don't hear a prosodic voice, yet a low monotone. The vagus takes the brake off the heart to prepare either the fight or flight reaction. And when that system comes up short and our life is in danger, the vegetative vagus stands up for itself and we lose consciousness.

Since the savvy vagus controls heartrate and breathing, respiratory sinus arrhythmia (RSA) measures vagal tone. RSA happens as the pulse accelerates while breathing in and backs off when breathing out. This inconstancy depicts a sound heart.

More noteworthy RSA improvements the quiet physiology of the savvy vagus and supports affiliative practices like eye to eye contact, tuning in, prosody and compliance. These features assist us with recognizing whether we are safe and, assuming this is the case, bolsters ideal learning practices.

In synopsis, the polyvagal hypothesis is multi-leveled: the more modern myelinated vagus restrains thoughtful barriers which hinder unmyelinated immobilization safeguards.

Messaging interferes with the "neural activities" of eye to eye correspondence so important to grounding our mammalian sensory system. Absence of training prevents these guidelines of commitment. Lose the telephone.

MINDFULNESS EXERCISE

Before the mission begins, do you have a moment to sit down, close your eyes, and focus your attention? Do you guarantee that you have 100 percent of yourself involved in the task? When you rest, do you take a moment to be grateful for your surroundings?

Mindfulness is exactly that: spend your time and effort paying attention to what you are doing and what is happening around you. Many of us jump from task to mission or set fire to one another without paying attention to what is going on around us. We have fallen into the head so much that we pay attention to a task and give it the full attention we receive on its back, it seems like a waste of time and effort to do it. Many health professionals, myself included, are to blame. We go from patient to patient or on an appointment, forgetting or not paying our full attention to the fact that one has our trust and decisions regarding one's health and life. Becoming a functioning physician gives me a chance to influence the lives of my patients in a positive and profound way so that I am more aware of the attention I can give to each patient. Before you bring the next patient, it takes a few minutes to review my notes, remove any distractions from my surroundings, and clear the tasks clearly with other things. In doing so, I take a moment to remind each patient that I trust them to achieve their health and life goals. The exercise included means maximizing each task with 100% of your attention on that task. This means taking in your surroundings, becoming aware of everything that came at this exact moment and being grateful to you. The ability to practice vigilance may not occur when we feel stressed, insecure, and painful. Our sympathetic nervous system tends to get our attention and prevent us from focusing on what we do. When you are really monitoring the whole day, focus on your breath and how you can accomplish each task. This alters the balance towards the parasympathetic nervous system and allows the VN to do its job. Taking on one task means doing one thing at the same time with full attention and finishing it before moving on to the next task. Eating with a spirit allows you to feel satisfied and not eat. Mindfulness relaxation makes you feel more comfortable and rejuvenated than you imagine. All of these require that the vagus nerve be active and involved because we must be able to trust it so that our bodies can rest, soothe, and recover. Multitasking is the exact opposite of alarm. Recognizing what I do, eat, and feel as each task undergoes one of the most positive changes I have made in my life is the first reason why my health aspect is so much more positive. It has been a major needle engine for a host of others around me and me, and I am sure that it can make profoundly positive changes in your life as well.

Meditate

Meditation is similar to the practice of mindfulness. It is the art of drawing your breath and teaching your attention not to follow all thoughts that arise in your mind. Our brains are designed. We are thinking and forming genuinely dynamic connections between our thoughts and actions. Meditation teaches us to listen to our hearts and focus our breath and learns to become observers of our thoughts instead of the victims of their floods. Instead of discussing many ways of meditating, I want to discuss the benefits. Heart rate studies have shown that meditation has important positive benefits on the function of the vagus nerve since, during meditation, our attention is directed to our breath. There are many different types of meditation, but those that focus on breathing are usually best at improving HRV levels. These include Breathing Meditation, Kindness Meditation, Vipassana, and Mindfulness Meditation.

One interesting piece of information I discovered during my research is that HRV showed improvement only in patients who did not classify as perfection. In the International Journal of Psychophysiology, a study by Azzam et al. It was found that control patients were more likely to have positive changes in HRV levels compared to those who identified themselves as perfection. Basically, "idealists" are focused on meditation fully or on the right path so that they do not allow themselves to relax and benefit from the practice itself. One of the most common things I hear when I ask my patients about meditation is that they are "unable to do it properly." This ideal attitude is exactly what prevents them from receiving benefits. If you practice meditation without any predictions or suggested notions about the "right way" to do so, it is easier to use this practice.

For starters, I recommend voice-guided meditations on YouTube or through an app on your phone. I recommend Headspace, Oprah Winfrey and Deepak Chopra and Meditation for 21 Days to Try, Calm and Insight Timer. For those who want to get feedback on practicing meditation, Heart's Inner Balance is a great tool to help you determine if you have entered a compatibility state, which is measured by heart rate. Another tool for those interested in getting first information is Muse, a meditation headband that measures brainwave activity and gives you real-time voice feedback. These are additional tools and are not necessarily practice, but they can be a good investment for those who usually seek perfection.

Laugh And Social Networks

If you know that laughing can improve your health, will you do much? I remember the last time I had a good laugh session with friends. Have you been happy in the next few hours? Do you sleep better that night? Are you expecting to wake up this morning?

Ongoing research often shows that laughter and yoga can be very effective in improving mood swings and heart rate. We tend to use our diaphragm when we vigorously laugh and enjoy it, so we practice our ability to control our breathing rate and ensure that we can normalize our breathing. This is the practice of the vagus nerve. Regular running is a great and very fun way to improve vagus nerve function. I watch funny videos or go to comedy programs when I feel as social as possible, and enjoy the health benefits of laughter. Laughing yoga classes in your community, meeting friends regularly to share fun stories, and playing comedy are all things great options for more laughs. Social engagement is directly linked to this because we can possibly laugh out loud when we are in the presence of others, especially friends and family. Social engagement is one of the biggest determinants of health and can be more important than the foods you eat. People want to be around other people. When we feel lonely and separated from others, our mood and health are negatively affected. We tend to enjoy the company of others and prefer to talk to real people. When we are around others, we tend to laugh more, laugh more, and feel more comfortable. We feel even better when we spend time with people who share our values with them. I recently took my family to the Living Proof Team Retreat in Minnesota, which was a great experience. Those beautiful natural environments and surroundings were combined with spending time with team members who share the same values as I do. We were taken care of by the team at Point Retreat, another wonderful group of individuals who appraise people for bringing a healthier and happier life. By the end of the trip, we were all very happy and comfortable, regardless of the travel pressure. If you feel single, feel, or just offline, look for a way to spend time with others and connect with people who share the same values with yourself. If fitness is important, then you can go to the gym or share a yoga lesson with friends. If communication is important to you, join the Toastmasters group, and practice your public speaking skills with supportive people who share the same thinking. If you value time with others, go to a movie or a meal with friends so you can talk and have fun. There are 7 billion people on the planet and many activities and interactions that allow you to connect with these people.

It is believed that as we age, we will laugh less, but the healthiest people I know will laugh more. In the blue regions, the regions with the highest rates of life worldwide (with many people over 100 years old still being physically active), social cohesion is a common theme.

So enjoy the social experience with those around you, meet new people, share funny stories, and laugh as loud as you can. Doctor ordered!

Listen To Good Songs

Are you not really satisfied after listening to good music and singing? This is because your body is already feeling comfortable and able to recover during and after this time. It is the same reason why we enter our favorite texts when we sit in our cars or walk-in traffic. A 2010 study by Chuang et al. Cancer patients who participated in a two-hour music therapy session that included singing, listening, learning, and music performance significantly increased heart rate measures and thereby increased vagus and parasympathetic nerve activity. Another study was written by Lynn et al. In 2014, HRV was used to show that Mozart music could improve parasympathetic nerve function. Much of this research was concluded with children diagnosed with epilepsy, a common seizure disorder. Listen to Mozart's music, especially Mozart's "K.448" sonata for two pianos, has shown a decrease in the frequency of strings and changes in the brain.

Next time you sit in traffic and feel nervous because you are late for a meeting or work, play some good music and let your body move and sing along. You will inevitably feel more relaxed and less stressed and continue at the same time. When you're at home and feeling comfortable, Mozart will play in the background and see what you feel next.

Smart Food Choice

As research slowly becomes clearer, we discover that there are foods that can have a negative impact on our cellular and digestive health and are more likely to increase inflammation levels. As discussed in most of these choices are highly processed foods, foods contaminated with antibiotics, hormones, herbicides and pesticides, and genetically modified foods. Avoiding these foods is important to reduce the risk of damage to the intestinal pollution, liver detoxification system, and the health of each of our cells. When I choose healthy and smart food, I recommend locally grown organic fruits and vegetables; lean chicken and eggs. Lean and grass-fed beef. Non-GMO cereals such as rice and quinoa; Organic nuts and seeds. For the majority of people, a green, clean, and gentle diet of healthy fats and nutrients that are processed as little as possible is the best place to start. To learn more about food choices, I recommend reading foods: Which one should I eat? Dr. Mark Hyman. Follow its protocol for four weeks, then add one food at a time. Remember that your diet is tailored to your needs and preferences. Vegetarian diets, autoimmune plants, pyto-ketones are useful, but nutrition should be appropriate for what you need. Remember that green, clean, and slim are my three rules when shopping at a grocery store or farm.

If you are looking for the specific enhancement of the function of the vagus nerve, foods with nutrients to help produce ACh are necessary. Acetylcholine is the major neurotransmitter used by the VN, and low levels may contribute to suboptimal vagus nerve activity and signaling. Nutrients necessary to enable the production of choline-rich ACh, such as egg yolk, high-quality organic cooked meats such as meat liver, chicken and turkey, and soy lecithin, a common food additive. Another effective tool to use to improve the function of the vagus nerve is to give it a rest - literally, allow your vagus nerve to take some time. Intermittent fasting and time-limited eating are effective tools to improve heart rate. This is a tool I personally used to balance sugar levels, improve energy levels, and reduce the amount of stress on my body. Intermittent fasting has been shown to increase HRV, a sign that vagus nerve function has improved, and health is improving in the long run.

For intermittent fasting or time-limited eating, limit your eating to a window of six to eight hours while you awake. For example, you can limit the intake of calories at breakfast, thus reducing the amount of sugar in the blood in the early day, and eating the first meal. Personally, I take two meals daily, at noon and 8:00 am, while I take amino acid powder every morning to make sure my cells have the tools they need to function optimally.

WHAT CAUSES INFLAMMATION OF THE VAGUS NERVE?

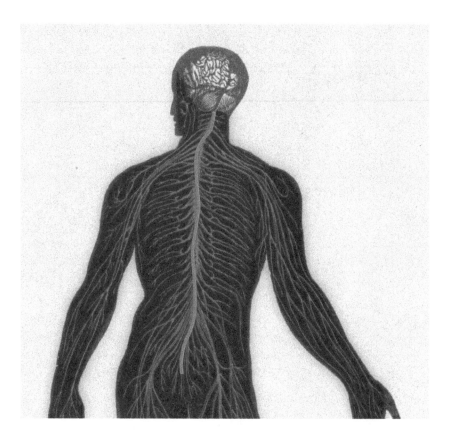

We have already observed that the vagus nerve is a delicate part of your body. Stimulation and stress to the nerve may lead to various health complications. In this section, we will be focusing on the causes of damage to the vagus nerve. As we have already seen, a damaged vagus nerve can be dangerous and can lead to some conditions that are beyond your control. To avoid getting to such a situation, you need to start providing the right care for your nerve. You are responsible for whatever happens to your nerve since you are the only person in a position to provide the right care.

Before we look at the inflammation of the vagus nerve, we should first try to understand what inflammation means. In simple terms, inflammation is the response of the body when fighting against infections or injuries that may be harmful. When any tissue of the body is attacked or injured, the body will naturally attempt to heal itself. This happens through a process in which the body releases chemicals that trigger a response from your immune system.

The process involves the release of antibodies and chemicals to the injured region. The region also experiences increased blood flow. The process may last a few hours or days. Chronic inflammation is a case where the entire process continues for long. This means that your body has to stay in a constant state of alert.

Although this definition of inflammation may sound like a good thing, inflammation may have a lot of side effects. You have probably had an open wound and observed the healing process. The inflammation stage usually leads to drying up of the wound. This leaves the skin in a dry and cracked state. At this stage, the wound may be itchy and very sensitive. This is the same case that happens to all our body parts. When the cells are injured or attacked by toxins, the body naturally tries to repair the damage. The efforts to repair the damage often lead to inflammation.

Inflammation of any internal body part will always lead to painful experiences. The same case applies to the vagus nerve. The vagus nerve may experience chronic inflammation. When your nerve undergoes inflammation, you may suffer pain just like any other part of the body. It is, therefore, important to protect your vagus nerve from chronic inflammation or any causes of the same. Prolonged inflammation has also been associated with various deadly diseases, including cancer. If there is a way you could avoid the inflammatory effects on the vagus nerve, it is advisable to take the right measures to stop it even before it starts.

There are several causes of inflammation of the vagus nerve.

- Untreated cases of acute inflammation, such as an infection or injury: There are many times when the vagus nerve may suffer infection. It is common for the nerve to be affected even by simple cold infections. Given that the vagus nerve spreads throughout the body, it is easily affected by injuries and infections that affect the other parts of the body. These infections should be treated early and be dealt with completely. If infections are not treated, they may cause inflammation of the vagus nerve later on.
- An Autoimmune Disorder: It is also possible for your vagus nerve to suffer inflammation due to immune disorders. Given that the nerve is a central part of the body processes, any immune disorder may easily attack the

nerve. Immune disorders occur when foreign materials get into the body or due to genetic complications. In either case, such immune disorders can easily lead to complications, including chronic infections and vagus nerve inflammation.

- Long-Term Exposure to Irritants: One of the most common causes of internal inflammation is exposure to irritants. People who work in toxic environments may be victims of vagus nerve inflammation. For instance, if you breathe polluted air that is filled with industrial chemicals at your workplace, you are likely to suffer chronic inflammation. This calls for self-protection from such harmful environments. Even if you have to work in an environment that is potentially dangerous to your health, make sure you wear protective gear. The vagus nerve extends to the heart and the lungs. It can be traced to your throat and the ears. This means that it is exposed to toxins that come into your body through food or air. If you breath toxic air, you may easily damage the vagus nerve. The same case applies to the foods you eat. You are responsible for ensuring that you do not get in toxic content that may affect your health or your vagus nerve in any way.

With that said, it is also important to understand that chronic inflammation cases are reported on a daily basis. Some of the underlying causes of inflammation are not clearly known. The fact that you work in a chemical industry does not necessarily guarantee that you will suffer vagus nerve inflammation.

Other factors that may lead to vagus nerve inflammation include.

- Smoking: Smoking is one of the activities that directly impact your vagus nerve. Given that cigarettes have different toxins, the continuous exposure of your nerve to these chemicals may lead to damage or inflammation. This is one of the obvious causes of cancer. As we have mentioned, sometimes the inflammation cases may directly result in cancer. It only makes sense that a person who smokes on a daily basis is likely to suffer chronic inflammation and even suffer from cancer.

- Alcohol: Another major cause of vagus nerve inflammation is alcohol. It is a fact that alcohol destroys cells, both in the stomach and in your throat. The vagus nerve extends to your throat and the intestines. If you keep on taking alcohol, the vagus nerve is forced to continue working on a healing mechanism. This leads to inflammation of the vagus nerve. A person who takes alcohol for a long time may end up suffering chronic inflammation, even leading to cancer and arthritis in the long run. For you to protect your vagus nerve, you must regulate the amount of alcohol you take on a daily basis. It is also advisable to take diluted alcohol other than taking highly concentrated alcoholic drinks. The less the concentration, the safer it is to your vagus nerve.

Stimulation of Vagus Nerve

Vagus nerve can also be inflamed due to increased stimulation. While stimulation of the vagus nerve is something good that can help you stimulate the parasympathetic action, it can also be dangerous. If the nerve is overstimulated, the chances are that the pressure on the nerve may get excessive and lead to injuries. You must especially avoid means of vagus nerve stimulation that are not natural. Some of the artificial ways of vagus nerve stimulation that can lead to inflammation include:

PEMF

Pulsed Electromagnetic Field (PEMF) is a therapy that is often used to increase the heart rate and variability. This therapy is often used to stimulate the vagus nerve, prompting parasympathetic actions. While the use of PEMF is not harmful, continuous stimulation of the vagus nerve using this approach may lead to injuries, damage, or inflammation.

Most people use electromagnetic stimulators over the throat to naturally increase appetite. The same approach can also be used for self-stimulation and boosting bad moods. The fact that the pulsed gadget is applied directly to the brain, neck, or gut, makes it even more dangerous. This means that the devices used in the stimulation process have to come in direct contact with a person.

At times, you may be exposed to vagus nerve stimulating machines without knowing. Before you start using any electronic stimulation devices, try to understand the principles under which it operates. While a gadget may help you by stimulation your vagus nerve during the first few days, continued stimulation may be dangerous. Continued stimulation may lead to the inflammation of the vagus nerve, which may, in turn, be costly to treat.

Probiotics

We are living in an age where people are obsessed with living their lives according to the trends. In recent years, many people have shifted to the lifestyle of taking supplements and probiotics. As to whether probiotics are good for your health or not is a subject for another day. In this section, we only look at the effects of consuming probiotics on your vagus nerve. As it turns out, consuming probiotics for long may actually affect the vagus nerve negatively.

We have already established that the nervous system is connected to the brain through the vagus nerve. This means that messing with the vagus nerve messes up with the entire system. Recent studies show that there is an effect of the gut microbiota on the brain. In other words, the probiotics you consume may find their way to the brain and affect the nervous system in its entirety.

In one animal study on mice carried out by MIT, mice supplements were enriched with probiotics. The mice that consumed the supplements experienced a positive change in GABA receptors, which were mediated by the vagus nerve. GABA receptors are vital in the brain since they help regulate mood and provide a clear connection between the brain and vagus nerve stimulation. Continuous consumption of probiotics foods means that you may be stimulating your vagus nerve even without knowing. Continuous stimulation of your nerve through such artificial methods may have an effect on your vagus nerve, leading to damage or inflammation in the long run. As much as probiotics have shown positive health benefits, they are also very effective in stimulating the vagus nerve. There is time to stimulate the nerve. Do not get used to eating probiotics daily since it may only lead to overstimulation of the nerve.

Serotonin

Serotonin is a monoamine neurotransmitter that can be consumed artificially. Although the body is fully capable of producing its natural neurotransmitters, most people prefer boosting their mental clarity by consuming artificial serotonin. Research shows that consumption of serotonin may lead to the activation of the vagus nerve through various receptors, including 5HT1A, 5-HT3, 5-HT6, among others. However, there are some receptors that may lower the activity of the vagus nerve. For instance, serotonin through the 5-HT7 receptors does reduce the activation of the vagus nerve. In simple terms, serotonin offers a mixed bag of reactions for any individual who wishes to activate their vagus nerve. This mixed outcome poses a big danger to the vagus nerve. When taking serotonin, you must be sure of the type of receptors you are targeting. The serotonin that activates the vagus nerve may still lead to inflammation. Continuous activation of the vagus nerve through artificial means only builds pressure on the nerve. When your vagus nerve is under pressure, it is likely to suffer injuries or get damaged. The final outcome of the injuries or damage includes inflammation. In case the vagus nerve is damaged, you have to use counteraction to reduce the inflammation caused by the natural healing mechanisms. It is recommended for those who take serotonin to use the 5-HTP for the purpose of increasing serotonin. However, you should take your supplements over a long period with a clear distribution of the injection sessions.

Body Stress and Vagus Nerve

Stress is a natural way of reaction to change that the body has to go through. A person is stressed when they face conflicting thoughts or when they feel threatened. If you are in a situation where you feel that your life is in danger, you are likely to experience stress. Stress is accompanied by varied physical, emotional, and mental responses. When you are afraid of something or worried about something, the body will prompt certain actions to take place naturally.

Although stress is a normal part of life, it brings varied ups and downs. It is not possible to take care of your nerves if you are constantly afraid. As a matter of fact, any time stress kicks in, and you should let the nervous system take full control. You may experience stress from your thoughts, your body, or from the environment. In either case, the vagus nerve will directly be affected.

As we have already mentioned above, any activity that leads to either direct or indirect stimulation of the vagus nerve may affect its health. If you are constantly stressed, the chances are that you may constantly keep on hurting your vagus nerve. We have seen that chronic inflammation only occurs after a long time of natural rehabilitation. If the body keeps on trying to rehabilitate worn-out tissues due to injuries, it will eventually lead to inflammation. The same case applies to stress. If you constantly experience stress, you are likely to stimulate the vagus nerve to such an extent that it is impossible to recover. But how exactly does body stress relate to the vagus nerve?

Any time you are under stress, you suffer from anxiety or panic attacks. Although the symptoms of either anxiety or panic attacks are not visible, it is clear that people who suffer stress may experience some form of anxiety. The brain is programmed to respond to such stressful situations by producing CRF hormones. Although the brain naturally produces such hormones, stressful situations lead to increased production of the hormones. The CRFs travel through the hypothalamus to the pituitary glands, where they cause the release of another hormone, known as ACTH. This hormone consequently travels through the bloodstream to the adrenal glands. This leads to the stimulation of cortisol and adrenal reaction, which helps protect the boy from stress. As you can see, this process of stress protection is long and directly affects your vagus nerve. When we are suffering from stress, we are likely to get deep into a state of depression if the vagus nerve and the brain get overwhelmed.

Stress and depression have all been linked with inflammatory brain response. In other words, the process of responding to stress puts the brain under extreme pressure, leading to injuries and inflammation. In other cases, the same applies to the vagus nerve. As the nerve is exposed to the stress of trying to deal with the anxious situation, it is common for the nerve to experience injuries. Such injuries attract the natural healing process of the body, which eventually results in inflammation. Even though the body naturally fights injuries, continued stress can lead to continued production of hormones, which eventually leads to actions that may cause stress to the vagus nerve.

Chronic stress can also lead to an increase in the production of glutamate in the brain. The production of glutamate may directly affect the brain and, as a result, affect the vagus nerve. For instance, glutamate is a neurotransmitter that causes migraines and depression when produced in excess. When you are under stress, it is common for the brain to initiate the production of this neurotransmitter. To protect yourself from such conditions and to ensure that you protect your vagus nerve from any damage, ensure that you reduce stressful moments in your life. There are many ways of dealing with stress, including meditation, singing, dancing, among others. Such options will help you deal with stress and reduce the pressure on your brain. By acting to reduce pressure on your head, you act to protect the brain and the vagus nerve as a whole.

In one research conducted by medical students from Ohio State University, it was revealed that when certain animals are put under excess pressure, they react by producing high levels of cortisol. The high level of cortisol produced tries to reduce the volume of the hippocampus. The fact that a person is under pressure only means that they reduce their chances of having a sober brain. If you are struggling with stress, the chances are that you may not be able to concentrate or keep memories. It is important to ensure that you reduce your levels of stress so that you concentrate on other aspects of life. If you do not pay much attention to your health and try to reduce the stress associated with your life situations, the chances are that you may end up living a life that painful.

All the factors that affect your brain are also impactful to your vagus nerve. Stress does not only affect your brain, but it also affects your nervous system. The vagus nerve may completely fail if you keep on undergoing episodes of stress on a daily basis. The inflammation of the vagus nerve may further lead to other health complications. Inflammation means that the nerve is not functioning to the maximum. A simple problem, such as inflammation, may lead to digestive and hearing problems. If the case advances, the entire vagus nerve may be affected and hence affect the autonomic nervous system.

Blood Pressure and Heart Rate

Another factor that may lead to the inflammation of the vagus nerve is blood pressure. The human body is designed to maintain a certain level of blood flow. This means that there must be signal transmission from the heart to the brain that coordinates the blood flow. The flow of the blood depends on the heart rate and the constriction of blood vessels. If blood vessels are constricted, the heart will be forced to pump the blood a lot faster so as to achieve equal distribution of blood to all body parts. In the same way, if the blood vessels are lost, the heart rate has to reduce to some extent. The vagus nerve is at the center of all the operations that affect the functioning of the heart.

Vagus nerve stimulation devices have been used for various medical purposes for more than 30 years. These devices are either implanted or used externally. Some of the common implants are devices that range in 1 to 3.5 mA. These devices are mainly designed to influence heart rate and blood pressure. Some of the diseases that these devices aim to control include epilepsy and heart diseases. With that said, it is evident that stimulation of the vagus nerve has a significant effect on the blood pressure and heart rate.

Research shows that most of the devices used in vagus nerve stimulation, either use mechanical pressure application or automated electromagnetic waves. In the early 1800s, the data collected from such devices was vital in evaluating the overall health of the vagus nerve. Data such as the Electrocardiogram

(ECG), heart rate (HR), and blood pressure (BP) were all evaluated. However, modern-day medical applications focus tends to be on the performance of the device rather than the wellbeing of the nerve. Over the years, most device manufacturers have opted to design invasive devices that do not give out data as it was initially. This does not mean that the devices used for vagus nerve stimulation are defective in any way. The main concern would be a case where the device was causing overstimulation, resulting in fatigue and injuries to the nerve.

It is recommended to use the non-invasive vagus nerve gadgets. Wearables such as the hand and thump pressure tools are much safer. Today, some manufacturers are reverting to the traditional options of belt and hand pressure. In either case, you must ensure that the gadget you chose to use has been approved and received a clean bill of health. Understanding that any stimulating device is only supposed to help you enhance activities that are already taking place will also help you understand that overstimulation may mess up with the natural processes. The human body is made to run naturally and provide internal solutions to internal problems. This explains why the vagus nerve has to defend itself from injuries. In the case of an injury, the nerve must initiate a process of self-recovery. In this process of recovery, the injuries caused to the body or to the nerves must be resolved.

If you choose to use a device that regulates your blood pressure, you must ensure that it does not go beyond the required. Overstimulation of the vagus nerve will obviously lead to excessive production of some enzymes. The parasympathetic activities of the nerve are awakened during a moment when the body should be acting in the opposite direction. Although the ultimate result of reducing heart rate may be achieved, it is still expensive and painful to experience some complications associated with the stimulation. If you want to stimulate your vagus nerve for the sake of reducing blood pressure and heart rate, only do it selectively. It should not be something you do daily.

DISORDERS ASSOCIATED WITH VAGUS NERVE MALFUNCTION

P oor vagal activity has significant health implications. The vagal pathway that connects the brain to organs in the body regulates physiological processes that are carried out by the heart, lungs, gut, liver, and other vital body organs. Through the vagus pathway, organs regularly send signals to the brain. This communication enables your brain to maintain the status quo when things are going well or trigger an adjustment when organ functions are being interfered with.

The net effect of this is that proper function and optimum health are dependent on the proper function of the vagus nerve. Your brain and organs depend on your vagal pathways to regulate processes like:

- Inflammation responses
- Anxiety and fight-or-flight responses
- Hunger hormones and food intake
- Immune responses

The vagus nerve is the link through which the enteric nervous system, that regulates the function of the gastrointestinal tract, communicates with the central nervous system. The central nervous system and enteric nervous system work together in the regulation of peristalsis, immune functions, and blood flow. This means that how well the vagus nerve is functioning will determine the efficacy of the brain-gut axis communication. This ultimately has an effect on everything from stress levels to heart rate to digestion to weight gain.

Symptoms of Vagus Nerve Dysfunction

Due to the importance of vagal activity in maintaining homeostasis in the body, when vagus nerve function is disrupted, there are inevitable impacts on our health and well-being. Vagus nerve disorders can be caused by a myriad of factors including;

- inflammation
- infections
- chronic stress
- certain diseases
- certain medications

Poor vagal activity will lead to interruption of all processes that depend on a rest and relaxed state in the body to function properly, including sleeping, heart rate regulation, breathing, and digestion. Poor vagal functioning can also affect neuronal activity in the brain and cause inflammation and neurodegeneration.

Some of the symptoms that point to poor vagal activity are;

Gastroparesis

This condition affects the ability of the stomach to empty itself by affecting the contractions that move food along the digestive tract. This condition can result in bloating, blood sugar fluctuations, vomiting, loss of appetite, or abdominal pain.

Vasovagal Syncope

Extreme stress factors such as exposure to extreme temperatures or even fear can result in an overreaction from the vagus nerve. This reaction occurs when the vagus nerve is overstimulated and results in a marked reduction of the heart rate and blood pressure. When this happens, the individual faints, which is characterized by a temporary loss of consciousness.

Chronic Fatigue

Fatigue is the feeling of physical and mental exhaustion and burn out. Typically, fatigue will manifest as a general lack of motivation and energy. While it is quite natural to feel exhausted after a long day at work or following intense physical activity, chronic fatigue is characterized by a perpetual feeling of tiredness and general malaise that cannot be attributed to any one particular factor.

If you notice that you wake up tired or experience a sluggish feeling throughout the day, even when you are not doing anything physical exerting, you may be suffering from chronic fatigue. When the vagus nerve is unable to effectively inhibit the sympathetic fight or flight responses, the body remains in a constant state of agitation, meaning that you are unable to feel rested or relaxed because your vagus nerve is unable to trigger the rest and relaxed state.

Irritable Bowel Syndrome.

The vagus nerve plays a significant role in enabling digestive functions, and when it is not working properly, abdominal disorders are common symptoms. When the vagus nerve is functioning properly, it inhibits inflammation by shutting down sympathetic responses that are responsible for inflaming cells lining the digestive tract. In the absence of this intervention by the vagus nerve, the sympathetic responses become prolonged, leading to inflammation in the bowel.

Moreover, the vagus nerve has a role in stimulating the movement of food along the digestive tract through peristalsis. This means that when the vagus nerve is not working properly, the digestive functions will be impaired, and this is also an underlying cause for irritable bowel syndrome.

Chronic Stress and Anxiety.

One of the most significant roles of the vagus nerve is to restore the body to a relaxed state and facilitate self-soothing that ensures that we are not constantly agitated. When we are anxious or stresses, the nervous system responds to this by triggering the fight or flight response. Part of this response is the release of hormones such as adrenaline and cortisol. These hormones, in turn, result in agitation and effectively prevent us from being in a relaxed state.

When the vagus nerve is functioning properly, it will override this fight and flight response shutting down the release of adrenaline and cortisol. However, when vagal activity is impaired, these stress hormones are continuously released into the body resulting in chronic stress and anxiety.

Chronic Inflammation

Chronic inflammation is usually an indicator that the immune system is overstimulated, and as a result of its prolonged action, the body starts to attack its own cells causing chronic inflammation. When the vagus nerve is functioning properly, it can switch off the prolonged response of the immune system by preventing the secretion of the tumor necrosis factor and stimulating the release of acetylcholine. These two mechanisms, when initiated by the vagus nerve, are effective in inhibiting inflammation.

Acid Reflux

The hypersensitivity to acid reflux is referred to as heartburn. We have all, at some point, experienced that burning feeling in our throats after eating certain kinds of food. This burning sensation is typically our body's response to excessive acid in the digestive tract.

The vagus nerve plays a vital role in the communication between the gut and brain, and if this communication pathway is disrupted, the regulation of the gut can be impaired, which can result in the accumulation of acid and heartburn as a result.

Inflammation

Nature equips both animals and plants with self-defense mechanisms for the purposes of ensuring species survival and propagation. Without these mechanisms, every threat or possible danger would be fatal, and this would make it impossible to sustain life. Roses have thorns, porcupines have quills, and humans, of course, have the immune system.

Our internal defense mechanisms are facilitated by the nervous system in the form of the flight or fight responses, as well as the action of the immune system. Inflammation is one of the responses that is used by the immune system to combat tissue damage and injury that may be caused by pathogenic infection or physical injury.

We have all succumbed to infection at one point, or other, whether it's a common cold, flu, sore throat or more complicated infections, our ability to recover from these is dependent on the ability of the immune system to fight off the infection.

An inflammatory response is triggered by the immune system to aid in the healing of wounds or infections from pathogens or tissue damage. Inflammatory reactions such as swelling when you hurt yourself or redness of a wound or secretion of pus are a sign that the body is fighting the infection by mobilizing white blood cells to the site of infection. Without inflammation, healing of wounds, infections, and tissue damage would be impossible.

Inflammation can either be acute or chronic, depending on what caused it and how long it lasts. Acute inflammation is short term inflammation and may be caused by tonsillitis, physical damage such as cuts and scrapes on the skin, bronchitis, or a sore throat. Typically, these conditions will last for a few days or a week, so the inflammation is not prolonged.

Chronic inflammation, on the other hand, occurs when inflammation is prolonged and lasts for a long period of time, ranging from weeks to months or years. When inflammation is prolonged as in the case of chronic inflammation, it ceases to be a defense becomes and becomes an underlying cause for physical orders that characterized by the cells of the immune system attacking the body's own cells resulting in tissue and organ damage.

Some disorders that result from chronic inflammation include:

- Rheumatoid arthritis
- Periodontitis
- Tuberculosis
- Peptic ulcers
- Asthma

Chronic inflammation can result from an overactive immune system response to an infection, pathogens, or foreign antigen remaining in the body for extended periods or from pathogens that the body cannot break down. Chronic inflammation is usually slow in onset and lasts for a long time and may ultimately result in tissue death or scarring of connective tissue.

When our sympathetic responses are over-activated, or our immune system is overactive, causing it to affect the cells in our own bodies, the inflammation that results is usually prolonged and damaging to body tissues and organs. A protracted inflammatory response starts to cause self-harm to the body by targeting healthy cells in much the same way it would invading pathogens.

If the immune system is not inhibited effectively by the parasympathetic nervous system, chronic inflammation can cause disorders in tissues and organs and ultimately impact the physical and psychological health of the individual.

The Role of the Vagus Nerve in Regulating Inflammation

Autoimmune diseases such as rheumatoid arthritis occur when the body through the immune system starts attacking its own cells. The vagus nerve with its parasympathetic roles in the nervous system aids in inhibiting the effects of overactive immune responses such as chronic inflammation by detecting the presence of cytokines and the tumor necrosis factor that is produced by the immune system.

Once these compounds are detected, the vagus nerve signals the brain, and this signal initiates the production of anti-inflammatory neurotransmitters such as acetylcholine. The vagus nerve also acts through the splenic nerve to limit the release of the tumor necrosis factor by macrophages and in this way, is able to effectively inhibit inflammation in the body.

Physical Disorders

Hypertension

The force that your blood exerts on blood vessels is referred to as blood pressure. Hypertension refers to a state in which the blood pressure is elevated higher than what is ideal for good health. High blood pressure can cause various complications, including stroke, heart diseases, or even kidney failure. It is, therefore, important to ensure that we effectively manage our blood pressure to avoid health complications that may be fatal.

Hypertension has been linked to a lack of adequate physical activity, diet, and poor stress management. When a person is obese or overweight, the heart has to work harder to pump blood, which means that the pressure of the blood being pumped increases, and this creates stress and damage on arterial walls. Poor diet choices that cause thickening or obstruction of blood vessels also increase blood pressure and have adverse impacts on cardiovascular health.

Chronic stress is a major predisposing factor for hypertension. The vagus nerve has a significant impact on stress management, meaning it is equally effective in regulating blood pressure and reducing the chances of hypertension. When our fight or flight responses are activated by the sympathetic nervous system to enable us to deal with emotional or physical stresses, our vital organs are strained by the increased demand for energy in the body. In this stressed state, our heart rate increases, our rate of respiration equally goes up, and our digestive tract functions are inhibited.

If we remain in this state of agitation for lengthy periods, this additional stress on our major organs inevitably leads to health complications such as high blood pressure. When the vagus nerve, which is parasympathetic in nature, is activated, it mitigates the effects of the sympathetic responses by restoring the body to a state of rest and relaxation by slowing down the heart rate, dilating the bronchioles and stimulating digestive functions. The vagus nerve is, therefore, an important therapy for hypertension through regulation of the heart rate and playing a significant role in stress management.

Rheumatoid Arthritis

Rheumatoid arthritis is an autoimmune disorder that is caused by chronic inflammation. When a protracted inflammatory response causes tissue damage in the joints, it leads to rheumatoid arthritis, which manifests symptoms including; swollen joints, joint pain, the development of rheumatoid nodules, limited range of motion in the affected joint and in extreme cases may result in joint deformity.

Vagus nerve inhibition of cytokine production serves to reduce inflammation, and this has been found to be effective in providing symptomatic relief for rheumatoid arthritis patients. When inflammation is reduced, then the swelling in the joints and the pain can be significantly reduced, meaning that the patient can experience relief from the symptoms of rheumatoid arthritis.

Vagus nerve stimulation in Rheumatoid arthritis patients has been found to have a significant impact on the secretion of the tumor necrosis factor. When the tumor necrosis factor is actively being secreted, it causes inflammation, and thus by inhibiting its production, the vagus nerve is able to reduce the levels of inflammation in the body, which results in a reduction in the severity of rheumatoid arthritis.

Crohn's Disease

Crohn's disease and ulcerative colitis are characterized by the inflammation of the digestive tract. Crohn's disease leads to the development of symptoms such as abdominal pain, diarrhea, weight loss fatigue, and even malnutrition in extreme cases.

The development of Crohn's disease has been linked to factors such as malfunctioning of the immune system and genetics. Though most who suffer from Crohn's disease may not have a family history of the disease, genes have been found to play a role in increasing susceptibility to the disease. A protracted immune response to infections has also been found to be a possible cause for the development of Crohn's disease.

When you have a bacterial infection in the digestive tract, the immune response may be overstimulated, leading to chronic inflammation. In such a scenario, the immune cells will start attacking even the cells that form the inner lining of the digestive tract. When this happens, the damage to the cells lining the digestive tract is inevitable.

Vagus nerve stimulation is effective in relieving inflammation by inhibiting the effects of an overactive immune response. A non-drug therapy targeting the anti-inflammatory pathway of the Vagus nerve has been found to ease inflammatory systems in colitis and inflammation of the digestive tract. The high tumor necrosis factor characteristic in inflammatory bowel diseases can also be inhibited by the parasympathetic function of the vagus nerve.

The vagus nerve can prevent peripheral inflammation by initiating the release of glucocorticoids through the activation of the hypothalamic-pituitary-adrenal. Additionally, the release of Acetylcholine effectively inhibits the production of the tumor necrosis factor, which is a factor for inflammation.

Diabetes

The hormone insulin is a necessary component in the breakdown of glucose to provide energy to cells in the body. This means that when a person has low insulin levels or insulin insensitivity, the cells in the body are unable to access energy from glucose in the blood. This results in hyperglycemia or the presence of excess glucose in the blood, which is brought about by the lack of efficient breakdown of glucose. This condition where there are excess glucose levels in the blood is referred to as diabetes and can occur in two types;

Type 1 Diabetes

In type I diabetes, the immune system attacks cells in the pancreas, which in turn interferes and inhibits the production of the hormone insulin. Since insulin is required for the breakdown of blood sugar, once its production is repressed, it then results in an elevation of blood glucose levels because glucose is not being broken down effectively.

Type 2 Diabetes

Type 2 diabetes is mainly caused by the body's inability to use insulin efficiently due to insulin insensitivity or when the body does not produce sufficient amounts of insulin to breakdown blood glucose levels.

Stimulation of the vagus nerve can aid in regulating insulin production by inhibiting overactive immune responses that result in the destruction of the pancreatic cells that function in insulin production. While the immune system is crucial in preventing infections in the body, the overstimulation of the immune system results in the destruction of the body's own cells.

Initiating the parasympathetic responses of the vagus nerve by stimulating it can impede the production of the tumor necrosis factor, which causes inflammation. Additionally, by the production of acetylcholine neurotransmitter, the vagus nerve helps in regulating inflammation.

Gastroparesis

The normal function of the digestive tract requires that the food moves along the digestive tract so that digestion or food breakdown can take place. When food is moving along the digestive tract, nutrients can be extracted from the food and absorbed by the body, and waste products can be efficiently eliminated from the body. These processes are crucial for a healthy abdomen.

Gastroparesis occurs when this process is inhibited, and food does not move along the digestive tract as required. This condition is caused by the dysfunction of the vagus nerve. The muscles in our stomach rely on the vagus nerve to innervate them and facilitate the movement of food through peristalsis. If these muscles do not function properly, then food movement along the digestive tract is inhibited.

Gastroparesis is characterized by symptoms such as bloating, nausea and vomiting, loss of appetite, and weight loss. Gastroparesis makes control of blood sugar difficult and predisposes patients to the formation of obstructions in the stomach that prevent food from passing into the small intestine. Additionally, bacteria can easily grow when food ferments in the stomach.

Stimulation of the vagus nerve innervates the stomach muscles enabling movement of food along the digestive tract. Further, by keeping the body in a relaxed state, the vagus nerve creates a conducive environment for digestive processes, unlike sympathetic responses of fight or flight, which inhibit optimum digestive functions from taking place.

Mental Disorders

Alzheimer's

Neurodegenerative illnesses are triggered by the protracted activation of the microglia. This chronic activation creates a predisposition to degenerative diseases such as Alzheimer's and dementia. Alzheimer's is a cognitive disorder that is typically characterized by memory loss of memory, impairment of the cognitive ability, which ultimately leads to the progressive and gradual loss of behavioral and social engagement skills.

Alzheimer's causes systemic degeneration and death of brain cells. The net effect of this is the impairment of brain functions and cognitive abilities. Alzheimer's ultimately leads to dementia, which is a condition brought about by the decline in mental function that impairs the sufferer's ability to live and function normally. Alzheimer's presents as a progressive ailment starting with forgetfulness and memory loss and gradually resulting in the inability to perform even simple and straightforward tasks.

Our ability to perform simple physical tasks such as eating or bathing and cognitive functions such as memory, recognition of people and places, or operating machinery and tools is normally wired into our brains. This is why patients developing Alzheimer's will forget even their children's names or where they live and will be unable to do tasks that they were able to do before, such as driving. Deterioration of the brain cells inevitably causes us to lose our mental aptitude and erases most of what we know.

Alzheimer's is a distressing condition not only for a patient who slowly loses all notion of who they are but also for the family members who watch the gradual deterioration happen and the transformation of a person from an independent functional human being to a helpless person dependent on others. While there is no treatment that can cure Alzheimer's, there are therapies that are used to slow down the degeneration of brain cells.

Vagus nerve stimulation therapy can effectively inhibit the chronic microglia stimulation and thereby aid in slowing down of the neurodegeneration. Observations on the effect of vagus nerve stimulation on the microglia illustrate a morphological change that deters neurodegeneration in the brain cells. Microglia in patients with chronic inflammation shows fewer and shorter branches when compared to the microglia in a person with a healthy central nervous system where the parasympathetic responses of the vagal nervous system are able to mitigate overstimulation of the microglia.

<u>Epilepsy</u>

Epilepsy is a neurological disorder that is characterized by seizures that are triggered by abnormal brain activity. The abnormal brain activity interrupts the normal function of various organs which results in epileptic patients exhibiting the following symptoms;

- Uncontrollable jerking movements in the limbs
- Staring
- Confusion
- Loss of consciousness

Focal epileptic seizures are caused by abnormal activity in one part of the brain. These types of seizures may result in complete loss of consciousness where the patient becomes unresponsive to their environment, or they may not cause a lack of consciousness but cause involuntary jerking of limbs, dizziness, or alter smells and appearance of objects.

Generalized seizures result from abnormal brain activity in all parts of the brain. They can be in the form of;

- Petit mal seizures which normally affect children and tend to cause subtle body movements and may cause loss of consciousness
- Tonic seizures which affect muscles in the back, arms, and legs
- Atonic seizures typically cause loss of muscle control.
- Clonic seizures which affect the facial tissues, neck as well as the arms and manifest with jerking muscle movements during the seizure.
- Grand mal seizures can cause an abrupt loss of consciousness, jerking movements of the body, and in some cases, tongue biting.

The abnormal brain activity that brings about epileptic seizures may be due to other conditions such as stroke or head trauma. Infectious diseases that target the brain, such as meningitis and prenatal injury, can also result in seizures. Children with epilepsy may outgrow the condition as they grow older, while in some epileptic patients, lifelong treatment is necessary to control seizures.

Vagus nerve stimulation is a therapy used in the treatment of epilepsy that involves the use of a pulse generator to stimulate the nerve into calming and reducing abnormal brain activity, which causes seizures. The role of vagus nerve therapy in epilepsy is in reducing the intensity, frequency, and duration of seizures.

The calming effect of the vagus nerve serves to diminish and limit abnormal brain activity such that even when the epileptic seizures occur, they are mild and more manageable. While the vagus nerve stimulation therapy cannot cure epilepsy, it plays a significant role in managing seizures when used long term in conjunction with epileptic drugs.

INTRODUCTION CRANIAL NERVES AND THEIR FUNCTIONS

The cranial nerves are nerves that are in communication with the brain and go through the holes in the base of the skull in order to innervate different structures, in addition to the head and neck, for example if we refer to the gastric or vagus nerve, its area of Enervation includes viscera located in the mediastinum and in the abdominal cavity.

According to its emergency point on the surface of the brain, twelve pairs of nerves are distinguished.

From the physiological point of view, the cranial nerves can be divided into three groups or categories.

- Sensory or sensory nerves (olfactory, optical and auditory)
- Nerves engines (engine ocular   common,   pathetic, abducens, spinal, hypoglossal)
- Mixed or sensitive nerves - motor (trigeminal, facial, glossopharyngeal, pneumogastric).

In each cranial pair we can consider a real origin and an apparent one: Apparent

origin: it is the emergency site of the nerve on the surface of the brain mass.

Real or true origin: it is the site that gives rise to the nerve fibers that constitute the nerve.

In the case of the sensory or afferent nerves, their real origin corresponds to the peripheral nerve cells, which can be grouped together forming nodes attached to the nerve trunks, or be located in the sensory organs, for example the nostrils, eyes or ears. The motor or afferent nerves, begin in neuronal groups located inside the brain, which constitute its nucleus of origin.

Mixed nerves have two roots, one motor and one sensitive, each of which has its own real origin.

Some cranial nerves have vegetative fibers belonging to S. Parasypatic, this is the case of the nerves: m. common eye, facial, glossopharyngeal and pneumogastric.

These nerves, in addition to their motor sensory origin, have a central nucleus where their vegetative fibers originate.

I. Cranial Nerve: Olfactory Nerve

It is a sensory nerve that gives rise to the sense of smell.

Real origin: the olfactory nerve fibers originate in the bipolar cells of the olfactory mucosa or yellow spot, located in the upper portion of the nostrils.

These cells have ascending axons that constitute the olfactory nerve fillets.

Apparent origin: lower face of the olfactory bulb, located on the sieve plate of the ethmoid, on each side of the crista galli process.

Paths: nerve fibers from bipolar cells. They are found in several directions and then meet in 12 to 20 olfactory branches, which cross the sieve plate of the ethmoid and reach the lower face of the olfactory bulb.

In intimate contact with the olfactory nerves, there are a small pair of nerves called terminal nerves.

Ii.Cranial Nerve: Optic Nerve.

It is a sensory nerve that emerges from the eyeball; It is the nerve that allows us vision.

Real origin: originates in the layer of retinal ganglion cells. The axons of this ganglion cells, when meeting and going backwards, form the optic nerve.

Apparent origin: it is the anterior angle of the optic chiasma.

Travel and relationships: this nerve measures approximately 4 cm. In length, and goes up, back and inside.

The fourth segment is described in it.

First segment: intraocular. The axons of the retinal ganglion cells converge on the optic papilla : from there, the nerve pierces the superficial layers of the eye (sclera and choroid) at a site called the cribose area.

Second segment: intra orvitary. The nerve is comprised in a cone formed by the straight muscles of the eye and is immersed in the retroocular fat. At the apex of the orbit by the fibrous ring that provides insertion to the straight muscles (Zinn's ring).

In this segment the nerve is related above with the ophthalmic artery and outside with the ophthalmic ganglion.

Third segment: intracanacular. The nerve passes through the optic hole accompanied by the ophthalmic artery. At this site, fracture nerve injury that compromises the base of the skull and vertex of the orbit is common.

Fourth segment: intracranial. It measures 1 cm., and is between the optical hole and the chiasma. In this segment the nerve is located above the pituitary store and the sphenoid optic canal.

Iii.Cranial Pair: Common Eye Motor

It is a motor nerve that also has a constringent of vegetative fibers intended for the intrinsic muscles of the eye.

It innervates all the extrinsic muscles of the eye, exempt from the greater oblique and the external rectum; also, by its connection with the ophthalmic ganglion, it innervates the sphincter of the pupil and the ciliary muscle that are intraocular or intrinsic muscles.

Real origin

The fibers of this pair originate in two nuclei:

Somatomotor nucleus: located in the cerebral peduncles, at the level of the anterior quadrilateral terms and in front of the Silvio aqueduct.

Motor parasympathetic nucleus: it is the Edinger-Westphal nucleus or pupillary nucleus, which is located behind and inside the present. This is a photo motor and photocomputer core

Apparent origin

The nerve emerges in the groove of the common ocular motor. Located on the inner antero face of the corresponding cerebral peduncle.

Route and relationships

The common eye motor after emerging from the brain stem is directed outward up and forward. Passing through the posterior cerebral artery and the superior cerebellar artery then penetrates an external wall of the fleshy dome, placing itself above the optic and optic nerve. It exits the outer wall in the anterior portion of the cavernous sinus and enters the orbit through the sphenoid cleft, dividing into two terminal branches that cross the Zinn ring.

TERMINAL BRANCHES

- Upper terminal branch: Innervates the upper rectus muscle of the eye and the upper eyelid elevator.

- Lower terminal branch: innervates the internal rectum, the inferior oblique and the inferior rectum. It also gives a branch destined to the ophthalmic ciliary ganglion, which provides the parasympathetic fibers that regulate the pupillary sphincter through the short ciliary nerves.

Iv. Cranial Nerve: Pathetic Nerve Or Trochlear Nerve

It is an exclusively motor nerve that innervates only the greater oblique muscle of the eye. It has two peculiarities with respect to the other cranial nerves:

- It is the only nerve that emerges from the posterior aspect of the brain stem.
- It is the only cranial nerve that intersects its fibers inside the brainstem.

Real origin

In the nucleus located in the cerebral peduncle below the somatomotor nucleus of the common ocular motor nerve. The fibers that come from this core, before appearing on the surface intersect with those on the opposite side.

Apparent origin

Emerges on the back of the cerebral peduncles, on each side of the Vieussens valve frenulum.

Route and relationships

Surround the lateral faces of the cerebral peduncles and head forward, in the direction of the cavernous sinus. It penetrates the outer wall of said sinus, and is located at the beginning below the common ocular motor and above the ophthalmic. Then it enters the orbit through the sphenoid cleft and passes out of Zinn's ring.

Its terminal branch penetrates the greater oblique muscle of the eye, which it innervates.

V. Cranial Nerve: Trigeminal Nerve

Mixed nerve. It receives the sensitivity of the teguments of the previous two thirds of the skull, of the entire face, nostrils, orbital, oral cavity and its contents. In turn it is the motor nerve of the chewing muscles and some others.

Real

origin Sensitive origin:

The sensory fibers of this nerve are born in the Gasser ganglion, located at the apex of the anterosuperior face of the temporal crag. Said ganglion has an upper face, a lower face, an anteroexternal, convex edge, and an internal, concave, posterior border. The anteroexternal edge of the Gasser ganglion gives rise to fibers that constitute the ophthalmic, upper maxillary and sensory part of the lower maxillary nerve.

The fibers that start from the postero-internal edge of said ganglion form the sensitive root of the trigeminal, which is directed backwards and inwards to enter the protuberance and end in a long column of gray matter, called the trigeminal termination sensitive nucleus.

The trigeminal termination nucleus extends from the upper part of the posterior horn of the cervical medulla to the corresponding cerebral peduncle with a maximum thickness at the level of the protuberance.

This core has three levels: upper, middle and lower.

The inferior part or bulbomedular, constitutes the gelatinous nucleus and the fibers that synapse in this nucleus are in a predominant relationship (although not exclusively).

Motor origin:

Trigeminal motor fibers are born from two nuclei:

- Main or chewing core: It is located in the shell of the annular protuberance
- Accessory nucleus: It is located above the precedent, in the midbrain (cerebral peduncles).

Apparent origin

Emerges from the anteroinferior face of the annular protuberance, at the level of the middle cerebellar peduncles, by two roots: an external, thick root, which is sensitive, and another, thinner internal root, which is the motor root.

Route and relationships

The two roots are directed from the anterior inferior aspect of the bulge forward and outward towards the upper edge of the cliff.

The motor root is progressively located below the sensitive root.

Both roots cross the upper edge of the rock by the Gruber recess, and then the sensitive branch unfolds in a fan forming the triangular plexus that ends in the Gasser Ganglion.

The motor root slides below the sensitive root, passes below the Glaeer ganglion and then joins the lower maxillary branch.

In this way, the trigeminal nerve gives branches that are sensitive and a third that is mixed.

Terminal branches

It is the only cranial nerve that gives its terminal branches inside the skull.

1 - Willis ophthalmic nerve: sensitive

2 - Upper maxillary nerve: sensitive

3 - Lower maxillary nerve: sensitive motor

Each of these branches has an annexed ganglion:

1 - Ophthalmic nerve: it presents as an annex to the ciliary or ophthalmic ganglion, located within the orbit.

2 - Upper maxillary nerve: it is attached to the sphenopalatine ganglion, which is located in the peterigomaxillary fossa.

3 - Lower maxillary nerve: it has an attachment to the optic ganglion, located under the oval hole.

SAW. Cranial nerve: External ocular motor or abducens nerve

It is an exclusively motor nerve, destined for the internal rectus muscle of the eye.

Real origin: the external ocular motor nerve has its real origin in a protuberancial nucleus located below the floor of the fourth ventricle and that makes prominence in the ventricular floor giving rise to the eminence teres.

This nucleus is surrounded inside, behind and outside by the motor root of the facial nerve.

Apparent origin: the external ocular motor emerges from the bulboprotuberancial groove, on both sides of the blind hole.

Routes and relationships: from its apparent origin the MOE is moving forward, up and out; it penetrates into the interior of the cavernous sinus and travels it from the back forward in the company of the internal carotid artery. Then the nerve penetrates the orbit through the sphenoid cleft, through Zinn's ring.

The sixth cranial nerve does not emit any collateral branch and ends in the deep branch in the deep face of the external rectus muscle of the eye.

Vii. Cranial Nerve: Facial Nerve.

It is a mixed nerve: motor, sensory-sensory and vegetative organ.

It consists of two roots: a sensitive root called the Wrisberg intermediary nerve.

The facial itself has motor fibers destined to innervate the muscles of the mime, cutaneous neck, occipital, posterior digastric belly, stylohyoid and stirrup muscles.

The intermediate nerve of Wrisverg or VII º bis, picks up the sensitivity of the posterior part of the external auditory canal; This is the only sensitive territory of the facial and is called the Ramsay-Hunt area.

Real origin: somatomotor nucleus: it is located in the protuvedential shell, it borders the medulla oblongata. The fibers that are born from this nucleus, before emerging from the brainstem, surround the nucleus of the sixth pair, making prominence on the floor of the fourth venticle.

Sensory-sensory nucleus: this part of the nerve originates in the geniculate ganglion, located inside the temporal bone boulder.

The fibers that start from the geniculating ganglion, penetrate the spinal bulb to end in the upper part of a nucleus called the solitary fascicle (real termination nucleus of the sensory-sensory part of the facial).

Vegetative nucleus: they are two nuclei located in the protuberance, behind the motor nucleus.

- Lacrimomuconasal nucleus: its fibers stimulate the secretion of the lacrimal glands and nasal mucosa glands.
- Upper salivary nuclei: gives rise to the fibers that regulate the secretion of the submaxillary and sublingual glands.

Apparent origin: the VII cranial pair and the Wrisberg intermediary emerge from the protuberancial bulb groove in the area of the supraolivar pits, outside the VI th pair and ahead of the auditory nerve.

Route: from the protuberancial bulb groove, the two branches of the facial are directed upward and outward across the pontocerebellar angle in the company of the eighth pair, with which it is introduced into the internal auditory canal, accompanied by the internal auditory artery.

At the bottom of the internal auditory canal, the facial is located in the anterosuperior quadrant and penetrates the fallopian aqueduct through its entire length.

The nerve, like the aqueduct, has three segments:

- First segment or labyrinthine.
- Second segment or tympanic segment.
- Third segment or mastoid segment.

The facial nerve leaves the skull through the stylomastoid hole, located between the base of the mastoid process and the styloid process. It is then introduced into the parotid cell and in the thickness of the parotid gland it is divided into its terminal branches: facial cervical nerve and temporofacial nerve.

Collateral branches: Intrapetrose branches and extrapetrous branches are distinguished.

Intrapetrose branches

- Greater superficial petrosal nerve.
- Minor superficial petrosal nerve.
- Stirrup muscle nerve.
- Eardrum Rope
- Anastomic bouquet for the X th pair.
- Sensory branch of the external auditory canal.

Extrapetrous branches

- Anastomic bouquet for the X th pair.
- Posterior atrial nerve
- Digastric nerve.
- Lingual Bouquet

Terminal branches.

- Timerofacial nerve
- Cervicofacial nerve

Viii. Cranial Nerve: Auditory Nerve.

The auditory nerve, also called the statoacoustic nerve or vestibulo-cochlear nerve, is a sensory-sensory nerve that is related to hearing and balance. It is formed by two anatomically and physiologically different branches:

1st vestibular branch or balance nerve.

2nd Cochlear branch, in relation to hearing.

Real origin:

a) vestibular branch: the bodies of the origin neurons are found in the Scarpa ganglion (real origin). Their dentrites carry the balance receptor organs that are the utricule, the saccule and the semicircular conductors (superior, external and posterior).

From the Scarpa ganglion, the axons that form the vestibular branch leave, and go to the brain stem ending in the vestibular nuclear complex (nuclei of real termination), located in the bulb and bulge.

- Internal dorsal nucleus or Schwalbe.
- External or Delters dorsal nucleus.
- Core or Betcherew core.

b) Cochlear branch The real origin of this branch is the Corti ganglion or Spiral ganglion, located inside the membranous snail.

- Ventral cochlear nucleus.
- Dorsal cochlear nucleus.

Apparent origin: it is the bulboprotuverancial groove, outside the facial nerve and the Wrisberg intermediary.

Path and relationships: at the bottom of the internal auditory canal, both branches are in relation to the facial nerve, the Wrisberg intermediary and the internal auditory artery. From the internal auditory canal, the nerve is directed towards the lateral part of the bulboprotuverancial groove, passing through the pontocerebellar angle, where it is fundamentally related to the facial nerve.

Ix. Cranial Nerve: Glossopharyngeal Nerve.

The glossopharynx is a mixed nerve: sensory-sensory, motor and vegetative.

Function sensory-sensory: leads the overall sensibilidad of the pharynx and the posterior third of the lingual mucosa, tonsillar region and part of the veil of the palate.

As sensory nerve collects the gustatory stimuli of the posterior third of the tongue.

Motor function: innervates the muscles of the pharynx and veil of the palate.

Vegetative function: it contains parasympathetic fibers that innervate the parotid gland and the linguo-lavial mucous glands.

Royal Origin

- Motor origin: upper part of the ambiguous core located in the medulla.

- The middle and lower segments of this nucleus correspond to the motor origin of the pneumogastric and spinal respectively.
- Sensory-sensory origin: it is located in two ganglia.
- Andersch Ganglion
- Ehrenritter's Ganglion

Vegetative origin: the real origin of the vegetative fibers is located on the floor of the fourth ventricle, corresponding to the inferior salivary nucleus.

Apparent origin

The glossopharyngeal nerve emerges from the posterior collateral groove of the spinal bulb, above the pneumogastric and spinal.

Routes and relationships

The nerve exits the skull through the torn posterior hole behind the pneumogastric and spinal, from which it is separated by the jugular ligament. Then it descends through the retroestileo behavior of the maxillopharyngeal space to the base of the tongue where it ends.

1. Jacobson's nerve gives rise to six branches:

- Bouquet for the oval window
- Bouquet round window
- Tubal bouquet
- Carothotympathetic bouquet
- Major deep petrosal nerve

- Minor superficial petrosal nerve
- Nerve of the stylopharynx
- Nerve of the styglossus and glossostatine
- Tosilar or amigialine bouquet
- Pharyngeal bouquet
- Carotid bouquet
- Anastomotic bouquet for the facial (forms the Hallerr ansa)

Terminal branches

Upon reaching the base of the tongue, the glossopharyngeal is divided into numerous branches that expand into the mucosa, forming the lingual plexus.

X. Cranial Nerve: Pneumogastric Nerve

Mixed nerve: motor, sensitive and vegetative.

It is the one that has a more extensive innervation territory, since it includes viscera of the neck. Chest and abdomen.

Real origin

- Somatomayor origin: corresponds to the middle part of the ambiguous nucleus, below the motor origin of the glossopharyngeal.
- Somatosentive origin: it is found in two nodes located in the nerve path.
- Jugular ganglion: is located at the level of the posterior torn hole.
- Plexiform ganglion: it is more bulky than the previous one and is located below the base of the skull.

The neurons that form these ganglia, have dentritic extensions that are diminished by the territory of sensory enervation of this nerve (respiratory and digestive mucosa) and a central extension that penetrates the spinal bulb and ends in the nucleus of the solitary fascicle, located in the fourth ventricle floor (nucleus of real termination of somatosensitive fibers).

Vegetative origin: the vegetative fibers originate in two nuclei located under the floor of the fourth ventricle in the gray wing.

- Visceromotor nucleus: it is the dorsal nucleus of the vagus also called the cardioneumogastroenteric nucleus.
- Viscerosensitive nucleus: it is located outside the dorsal nucleus of the vagus.

Apparent origin

The pneumogastric emerges from the posterior collateral groove of the bulb, below the glossopharyngeal and above the spinal nerve.

Travel and relationships

Exit the skull through the torn posterior hole, positioned behind the glossopharyngeal and in front of the spinal. Then it descends through the backstage compartment of the maxillopharyngeal space.

In the neck, it is part of the high vasculonervious package, located in the dihedral angle that forms the internal carotid artery and the internal jugular vain. Below, it is part of the vasculonerviosa package under the neck, along with the primitive carotid and internal jugular vein.

In the thorax, the relationships are different for the right and left pneumogastric. The right pneumogastric passes in front of the right subclavian artery and behind the right bronchus. While the left descends in front of the arch of the aorta and behind the left bronchus.

In the lower part of the mediastinum, both pneumogastric are related to the esophagus; the right is located to the right and behind it, while the left vagus descends to the left and in front of the esophagus. In this way both pneumogastric will pass through the diaphragm through the esophageal hiatus, in intimate relationship with the esophagus.

In the abdomen, the left pneumogastric, applied on the anterior side of the esophagus, branches on the anterior face of the stomach. The right vagus follows the back of the stomach and is divided into two branches that end in the corresponding semilunar ganglion.

Collateral branches

- Cervical branches:
- Pharyngeal bouquets
- Cervical or superior cardiac nerve
- Upper laryngeal nerve
- Carotid bouquets
- Thoracic branches
- Inferior cardiac nerves

- Pulmolar Branches
- Esophageal bouquets
- Recurrent or inferior laryngeal nerve

ANXIETY AND VAGUS NERVE

Nervousness can be a genuine doozy; it's outlandishly muddled, profoundly close to home, and ridiculously difficult to foresee. There are times when we think our uneasiness is behind us—that we are at long last one stage ahead—yet then something movements and we are on our heels once more, battling to return to a position of harmony and quiet. We are on the whole understudies of our uneasiness and that is the reason seeing precisely how our sensory system functions—and what we can do to quiet it—can be staggeringly enabling.

In any case, what does quieting your sensory system truly mean? Numerous individuals would depict it as easing back the pulse, developing the breath, and loosening up various muscles—however, what associates these sensations to the mind? Indeed, enable us to acquaint you with the vagus nerve, the piece of the body that appears to clarify how our psyches control our bodies, how our bodies impact our brains and may give us the instruments we have to quiet them both.

Posttraumatic stress issue (PTSD) creates in people who have been presented to injury and subsequently languish trouble or utilitarian disability over in any event multi-month. Manifestations incorporate sentiments of re-encountering the horrendous mishap, keeping away from tokens of the injury, uplifted tension and excitement, and negative musings or emotions. Ongoing catastrophic events, mass shootings, psychological oppressor assaults and urban communities under attack add to the worldwide weight of PTSD which, as indicated by a recent report, influences 4–6% of the worldwide populace, although most of the injuries are identified with mishaps and sexual or physical savagery. Shockingly, there is no known fix, and flow medicines are not powerful for all patients. A PTSD psychopharmacology working gathering as of late distributed their accord proclamation calling for a quick activity to address the emergency in PTSD treatment, referring to three significant concerns. To start with, just two medications (sertraline and paroxetine) are endorsed by the US FDA for the treatment of PTSD. These meds decrease side effect seriousness however may not create a total reduction of side effects. The subsequent concern is identified with polypharmacy. PTSD patients are recommended prescriptions to address every one of their numerous extraordinary and assorted side effects including nervousness, trouble dozing, sexual brokenness, wretchedness and interminable torment, with lacking exact examinations of medication communications. The high comorbidity among PTSD and fixation gives further difficulties to pharmacotherapies. The third significant concern is the absence of headways in the treatment of PTSD; no new prescriptions have been endorsed since 2001.

Going past side effect alleviation, the 'best quality level' injury centred way to deal with treating PTSD pathology is introduction based treatment, where patients are presented to the tokens of the injury until they figure out how to connect these prompts with wellbeing. Although there is great proof for adequacy with this methodology, not all patients completely react to the treatment. Introduction treatment relies upon the way toward stifling the adapted dread memory, which is overwhelmed by another memory that creates through rehashed exposures. The patients with nervousness issue and PTSD show weaknesses in their capacity to quench adapted feelings of dread, which could add to the advancement of scatters and may meddle with the advancement in treatment. Since the memory of the injury isn't lost at the same time, rather, upgrades through treatment rely upon newly learned affiliations that rival horrible affiliations, the parity of the two recollections can move after some time, prompting backslide. Different difficulties incorporate the trouble in perceiving and smothering apprehension of every single moulded boost, and a high dropout rate, which isn't astonishing given that shirking is one of the indications of PTSD.

Numerous creature investigates labs have tried endeavours to create adjunctive medications to quicken or improve the impacts of presentation based treatments. Spearheading work did by Michael Davis demonstrated that organization of the psychological improving medication d-cycloserine before presenting rodents to unreinforced moulded signals upgraded annihilation, and he and his associates, therefore, deciphered the disclosure when they found that d-cycloserine likewise improved the impacts of presentation treatment in patients with explicit fears. In any case, aftereffects of studies evaluating the impacts of psychological enhancers as subordinates to presentation treatment are blended on account of PTSD. A conceivable clarification is that medications given before introduction treatment sessions risk fortifying negative affiliations if presentation produces nervousness. Anxiolytic medications have been attempted, in light of proof that these medications ought to improve decency and decrease the tension reaction during their introduction. Nonetheless, results show that anxiolytic medications don't improve the impacts of presentation treatment. One clarification is that the uneasiness reaction is required for accomplishment in introduction treatment since patients must learn not to fear their dread reaction. Then again, similarly as stress can improve the capacity of horrendous mishaps, the tension reaction may upgrade the combination of the termination memory. Predictable with this, anxiolytic medications will in general hinder memory combination. A perfect extra would take advantage of the systems that improve the union of horrendous recollections to advance elimination recollections that are similarly as solid, at the same time bypassing or maintaining a strategic distance from the aversive pressure reaction.

Developing proof proposes that vagus nerve incitement (VNS) might be a gainful extra to introduction based treatments through its blending explicit improvement of memory combination and neural versatility. Enthusiasm for the vagus nerve (the tenth cranial nerve) as a neuromodulator originates from a very long while of research demonstrating that the vagus nerve fills in as an extension between the fringe autonomic sensory system and the cerebrum. It flags the mind during times of elevated thoughtful movement, advancing quick stockpiling of recollections that are significant for endurance. As a major aspect of the parasympathetic sensory system, initiation of the vagus nerve neutralizes the thoughtful pressure reaction.

VNS upgrades the memory in rodents and people, proposing that blending VNS with an unreinforced introduction to adapted signals may improve the union of the elimination memory. Predictable with this theory, we found that VNS upgraded elimination of moulded dread in rodents. Broad proof shows that VNS advances neural versatility, particularly when it is combined with preparing, and this impact includes VNS regulation of the locus coeruleus noradrenergic framework. We have watched pliancy impacts in the termination related infralimbic prefrontal cortex – basolateral amygdala pathway in the wake of blending VNS with a presentation to unreinforced moulded prompts, proposing that VNS-improved elimination might be hearty, enduring, and less vulnerable to backslide. In an ongoing report, we found that VNS likewise improved termination of moulded dread in a rodent model of PTSD. These rodents express a considerable lot of the biomarkers and conduct phenotypes that are related to PTSD and, significantly, they are impervious to the elimination of moulded dread. We found that VNS organization during elimination sessions switched this termination disability and counteracted the arrival of dread. VNS-treated rodents likewise performed better on trial of tension, excitement, evasion, and social associations multi-week later, demonstrating that inversion of the elimination hindrance meant enhancements in other PTSD indications. Moreover, interminable, unpaired VNS, as is utilized in the treatment of epilepsy and despondency, improved execution on the Hamilton Anxiety Scale in certain patients with tension issue, and diminished uneasiness like conduct in rodents. The impacts of VNS on termination in our examinations are not seen when the VNS is managed 30 min to 1 h in the wake of preparing. In this way, VNS alone isn't adequate to decrease the dread reaction. These discoveries recommend that VNS may diminish nervousness, however, matching explicit pliancy and memory tweak is vital for elimination upgrade. Our ongoing, unpublished discoveries show that rodents are bound to investigate the open arms of a raised in addition to labyrinth following getting VNS, proposing that VNS produces an intense anxiolytic impact. Moreover, corticosterone levels expanded essentially in trick treated rodents following testing on the raised in addition to the labyrinth, however, such an expansion was not seen in VNS-treated rodents. This work ought to be imitated in different settings, yet it is an empowering initial move toward distinguishing an assistant treatment that may improve decency and adequacy in presentation based treatments.

The US FDA endorsed VNS as a strategy to forestall seizures in treatment-safe epilepsy patients in 1997, and 2000 for treatment-safe discouragement. The vagus nerve innervates the core of the single tract, which undertakings to the locus coeruleus and other limbic and forebrain cortical territories. VNS builds levels of monoamines in the cerebrum and the locus coeruleus assumes a job in VNS-initiated decrease of seizures. The current clinical routine with regards to VNS includes careful implantation of a terminal that is appended to one side cervical vagus nerve through an entry point in the neck. The cathode is associated with a lead that is burrowed under the skin to a heartbeat generator that is subcutaneously embedded in the chest. Careful inconveniences, for example, disease or vocal line impacts, happen in about 1% of patients. Less obtrusive ways to deal with animating the vagus nerve might be viable. In the nineteenth century, the nervous system specialist James Leonard Corning created gadgets to invigorate the vagus nerve transcutaneously, while compacting the carotid supply route, and he watched a lessening in the recurrence and span of seizures. These were not controlled examinations and Corning deserted the methodology because of reactions, for example, unsteadiness and syncope; be that as it may, transcutaneous VNS (t-VNS) has as of late recovered status as a clinical device. Noninvasive electrical incitement of the vagus can be controlled transcutaneously through the afferent auricular part of the nerve with cathodes cut to the concha district of the ear. With this t-VNS, the electrical boost, with a force that is above tangible location yet underneath the agony limit, is applied through the skin to the open field of the auricular branch. Blended outcomes were found in an ongoing report inspecting t-VNS consequences for the eradication of moulded dread in people and clinical research on the utilization of t-VNS is constrained, however, it is by all accounts sheltered and very much endured. Transcutaneous variants of VNS may give the advantages of VNS without the dangers of medical procedure; be that as it may, t-VNS isn't yet a setup treatment and assurance of its viability requires further examination.

VNS holds guarantee as an aide to introduction based treatments since it improves memory combination and advances synaptic pliancy while hosing the thoughtful pressure reaction. Although VNS has been utilized in people for more than two decades, the act of blending it with introduction treatment has not been tried in patients and numerous inquiries stay unanswered. 80% of the cervical filaments of the left vagus nerve are afferent tangible strands and preclinical examinations are right now in progress to inspect the general commitments of PNS versus CNS impacts of VNS. Singular contrasts in the nerve and excitement state may cause inconstancy in impacts in human patients. Recognizable proof of a solid biomarker for VNS impacts would be useful for redoing parameters in treatment crosswise over people, and it might be utilized to check the potential adequacy of less obtrusive strategies for invigorating the vagus nerve, for example, t-VNS. At last, it stays to be resolved whether VNS has an intense anxiolytic impact. As per our model, incitement of the vagus nerve sidesteps the thoughtful reaction to danger, while as yet advancing pliancy and quick union of enduring recollections. The job of the vagus nerve in the parasympathetic sensory system is to slow the thoughtful pressure reaction. Some proof shows that constant VNS decreases nervousness in people and rodents. On the off chance that VNS can quickly decrease uneasiness, this may, or may not be helpful for presentation based treatments. It might meddle with the chance to quench the dread of the dread reaction. Then again, it might rush advancement and improve consistency by cutting off the relationship between introduction to injury prompts and the moulded dread reaction during treatment. Studies are presently in progress to decide if diverse incitement parameters can be utilized to separate memory impacts of VNS from anxiolytic impacts.

During basic periods being developed, the cerebrum is more plastic than it is some time down the road. Be that as it may, when under strain, the grown-up cerebrum can adjust. Quickly put away, durable recollections of sincerely stimulating occasions are a case of strong neural pliancy that can be cultivated in the grown-up cerebrum. In 1890, William James expressed, "An encounter might be so energizing genuinely as nearly to leave a scar on the cerebral tissues". The neural pliancy that underlies horrible recollections can be versatile, decreasing the probability that perilous conduct will be rehashed. Once in awhile, awful recollections have maladaptive results, prompting tension or stress-related issue. We plan to bridle the capability of the vagus nerve to drive neural versatility during presentation treatment, while simultaneously intruding on the thoughtful battle or-flight reaction. On the off chance that fruitful, we will exploit instruments that exist to leave an enduring impact on the mind to mend the cerebral scars left by injury.

How is the vagus nerve affecting my wellbeing?

In 1921, a German physiologist previously found that animating the vagus nerve caused the pulse to back off by setting off the arrival of a substance he called Vagusstoff (vagus substance). It was later found that this substance was really acetylcholine—a significant synapse in our sensory system. From that point forward, scientists have found significantly increasingly about the vagus nerve and the job it plays in a significant number various infections and significant frameworks in the body. For instance, electrical incitement of this nerve has been appeared to decrease the pace of epileptic seizures and help with burdensome manifestations. Vagal tone—or how solid your vagus nerve is—can be associated with irritation, resistant framework guideline, digestion, and passionate guideline, which we would all be able to concur are entirely significant.

So what does the vagus nerve mean for psychological wellness? Low vagal tone is related with poor passionate and attentional guideline, aggravation, discouragement, and is even utilized as an estimation for an individual's affectability to push. Then, a solid vagal tone is related with the inverse: positive feelings and mental parity. A few investigations have even demonstrated that expanding vagal tone could be useful in treating fixation and certain longings. Knowing this, it may be time—to pay tribute to Mental Health Month—for us all to concentrate up on this significant piece of the body.

Would i be able to fortify my vagus nerve without anyone else?

Thinking about whether you can reinforce your vagal tone for better wellbeing? You're in karma! Numerous therapists, neuroscientists, and integrative wellbeing specialists state we can take advantage of the intensity of the vagus nerve to improve our emotional wellness. Christopher Bergland in Psychology Today composed that "Vagusstoff (acetylcholine) resembles a sedative that you can self-regulate essentially by taking moderate, profound diaphragmatic breaths." as it were, the vagus nerve has an inseparable tie to breathing—no big surprise associating with the breath is an establishing guideline in both yoga and contemplation. Be that as it may, other than breathing, there are a large group of various approaches to give your vagus nerve a truly necessary exercise. Here are five that will enable you to battle nervousness and weight on a neurobiological level.

1. Singing and music.

Research demonstrates that singing has an organically alleviating impact, which has an inseparable tie to the vagus nerve. This can be anything from a moderate mantra to reciting to belting out your top pick '90s melody.

2. Giggling.

In studies testing the impacts of vagus nerve incitement on kids with epilepsy, one of the symptoms is wild giggling. And keeping in mind that it is anything but an ideal reaction in a clinical setting, this shows chuckling is related with an expansion in vagal incitement. So chuckle and snicker frequently; there are such huge numbers of demonstrated advantages!

3. Irregular fasting.

A few examinations propose that fasting and dietary limitation can actuate the vagus nerve, and considering the various medical advantages of fasting, it's certainly something to consider.

4. Biofeedback.

Biofeedback, particularly pulse changeability biofeedback, is a stunning kind of innovation that works by showing a visual portrayal of what's going on inside the body. Along these lines, an individual can all the more likely comprehend the physiological impacts of profound breathing or unwinding strategies; the vagus nerve assumes a significant job in breathing guideline and pulse fluctuation, so this can be a fun method to practice it.

5. Cold presentation.

Studies demonstrate that cool presentation causes a move toward parasympathetic sensory system action, which as we probably am aware is adjusted by the vagus nerve. So in the event that you've never investigated the advantages of hot to cold showering, your vagus nerve could be a valid justification to begin.

6. Probiotics.

We definitely realize that the vagus nerve assumes a significant job in the gut-cerebrum pivot, however on account of science, we presently realize that gut microorganisms can really initiate the vagus nerve. As you can envision, this assumes a significant job in our cerebrum and conduct—on the off chance that you required another motivation to put resources into a viable probiotic.

IMPLEMENT A FEW LIFESTYLE CHANGES TO START INCREASING VAGAL NERVE HEALTH

- Cut down on alcohol consumption

Alcohol affects the Vagus nerve by spiking it into activity. This can cause erratic heartbeats, and if too much alcohol is consumed, it can and will end up damaging the nerve. A glass of wine at night may be fine, it could even have a positive effect on your heart. However, overdoing it leads to all sorts of problems, a lot of them may stem from the damage caused to the vagus nerve for alcoholism.

- Get more exercise

Exercise is essential for all parts of the body, not just the vagus nerve. But it is a great way to increase vagal tone and ensure the vagus nerve is functioning at its best. Dunking your face in cold water after strenuous exercises that have raised the body's temperature sets the vagus nerve in action.

- Get more sleep

It might seem that the answer to a lot of health problems is to get more sleep and there is a reason for that. Sleep is the time that your body gets to sort out problems, reset, and fight off nasty intruders into the system looking to do it harm. That is why, when there is a problem in the body, the vagus nerve will send signals to the brain to produce the hormones that make a person sleepy. While the body is at rest it is usually calm with minimal threat to it. This is the time when all the administration on the body begins. Kind of like what happens when a place shuts down for maintenance or how buildings are cleaned at night when no one is around. The next morning, you get to your office and it is all sparkling clean and ready for you to use.

The body has many working parts, which means it has a lot to do, including making sense of and storing away information you have taken in during the day. So, it needs a good 8 hours to get this done. Interruptions in the sleep pattern interrupt the body's functions. Soon, these escalate into bigger and bigger physical as well as mental issues.

It is also not just about getting enough sleep it is about getting enough quality sleep. This means making sure your sleeping environment is conducive to getting a good night's rest. In there is a section on how to make your sleeping environment sleep worthy.

Take note of how you sleep as well because sleep posture (yes, that is a thing), is really important to getting quality sleep, it also has an impact on the rest that your body receives.

- Eat more fiber

Eating more fiber is not just for people of advanced age who need digestive aid. It is for everyone. Fiber has been known to increase a hormone called GLP-1, and this hormone helps to slow down the emptying of the stomach to help you feel fuller longer. It is also a hormone that is important for helping communication between the vagus nerve and the brain.

This does not mean that you must go and eat copious amounts of fiber. It simply means that you should make sure you have at least the recommended daily amount that suits your body's needs.

• Add more seafood to your diet

Fish has always been said to be brain food, and that is because it is. A research study was done in 2014 that appeared in the American Journal of Preventive Medicine. The scientists found that fish increased grey matter in the brain. Particularly in the areas where Alzheimer's first tends to appear.

Eicosapentaenoic acid (EPA) and docosahexaenoic acid (DHA), both types of omega-3 fatty acids, are found in fish and help to stimulate the Vagus nerve and increase vagal tone. If you do not like fish, you can use fish oil supplements.

• Have intermittent bouts of fasting

The vagus nerve is a very busy nerve that is communicating with various parts of the body every single day, 24/7, 365 days a year. It is the go-between for communication between these parts and the central nervous system. One of its main functions is to regulate the digestive system. Fasting every now and then helps with a lot of things in the body like metabolism and regulating weight control. It also gives the vagus nerve a little rest so it can pay more attention to its other responsibilities. Intermittent fasting can also improve vagal tone.

- Sunlight exposure or Vitamin D supplements

Get more sunlight by spending time outside and soaking up the sun. Not too much sun though. What the sun does is gives us vitamin D, and vitamin D is very important for cardiovascular autonomic nerve function. As the vagus nerve is responsible for ensuring the heart rhythm is correct, vitamin D is essential for it to operate correctly.

- Meditate

Try and incorporate meditation into your day at least 2 to 3 times a week. Meditation has been known to slow down the heart rate and decrease blood pressure as it relieves stress and anxiety.

- Have a cold shower or splash your face with cold water often

Take a cold shower every now and then and splash cold water on your face at least once or twice a day. This stimulates most of the nerves and shocks the body into a response that stimulates the vagus nerve.

- Get a massage on a regular basis

Anything from a foot massage to a full body massage is good for stimulating the vagus nerve and getting the blood flowing to areas of your skin and body.

- Add zinc to your diet

Most people do not even realize they are zinc deficient, and it is crucial to the function of the vagus nerve. Try to supplement your diet with the recommended daily dose of zinc.

- Add serotonin to your diet

Serotonin has been known to activate various receptors that activate the vagus nerve. Speak to a pharmacist or medical professional about how to increase your serotonin and implement their suggestions into your lifestyle.

- Have probiotics on a regular basis

Gut health is important for the vagus nerve and keeping it healthy is a good way to increase vagal tone. Find a good probiotic by speaking to your pharmacist or medical advisor.

- Try pulsed electromagnetic field therapy

Although there are devices you can use by yourself at home, you do not want to overstimulate your vagus nerve. So, the use of these devices should be done under the strict supervision of your medical advisor. There have been some good outcomes with the use of these devices.

- Get out more and socialize

Believe it or not, socializing is a great way to increase vagal tone and get the vagus nerve stimulated. There are all sorts of benefits to mental health from socializing as humans are, by nature, social creatures. So, it stands to reason that limiting yourself or cutting off social contact altogether will be detrimental to our health.

Socializing helps build up our 'social-behavioral system' by fine-tuning it and making it more robust. Kind of like exercising your muscles builds up muscle tone, socializing helps build up a natural coping mechanism and thickens our hides so to speak.

- Smile and laugh often

If you are going to socialize more, then you should definitely make sure you smile and laugh more. There is a ton of research easily accessible to everyone about the health benefits of a smile and a full belly laugh. It not only has health benefits for the body, mind, and soul, it is also good for your social health. A person with a smile on their face is a lot more approachable and attractive.

Laughing and smiling are also a great way to increase vagal tone as they positively stimulate the vagus nerve.

- Dance and sing whenever you can

Dancing is a great feel-good way to stimulate the vagus nerve and music is a good way to get the energy flowing. Singing and humming vibrate and stimulate the vagus nerve into action. It is a good way to exercise the back of the throat and increase vagal tone. So, sing loud and strong as you dance like no one is watching you.

- Acupuncture

Try acupuncture as it is a great way to both stimulate and strengthen the vagus nerve. See or a bit more information on how acupuncture can help with the vagus nerve.

It is important to know that acupuncture can also overstimulate the vagus nerve, so it is very important to vet the acupuncturist well. Make sure they are experienced and have performed the procedure many times. It is also important to consult with your medical professional before trying it, especially if you have a preexisting condition.

Vagal Tone Measurement

A high heart rate variability usually means your vagal tone will be high too, this is measured by your heart rate and your breathing rate. The vagal tone can be increased by either having a medical device surgically inserted beneath your skin that sends electrical impulses to the vagus nerve or you can work on toning it naturally.

There is a device that can help you monitor and manage your heart rate variability (HRV) called the EmWave2. This device is also used by medical or scientific professionals in order to monitor and measure the vagal tone for both consulting and research purposes. If you are going to use any devices that monitor or have anything to do with the heart or blood pressure you should always seek advice from a trained, qualified medical professional first.

Stimulating the vagus nerve has been shown to be helpful in treating a few mental health issues and brain disorders.

Vagus Nerve Stimulation for Mental Health and Brain Conditions

- Anxiety

Anxiety is the feeling of having constant worries that escalate to a point where the person no longer feels in control of them. This leads to sheer panic and could bring about panic disorder.

People get anxious due to many different things, such as paying bills on time, worrying about their kids traveling on the school bus, having to get on a flight, and so on.

When a person is anxious, the body goes into its mobilization mode and triggers the fight or flight response. This releases various hormones into the system, and while a person is still anxious, the body continues to try and defend itself, so the parasympathetic system does not get a chance to bring the body back to a normal state.

With so many fight or flight hormones coursing through a person's veins, the mind is in a constant state of danger awareness so small things can seem like mountains. This can and usually does at some point lead to a full-blown panic attack.

The stimulation of the vagus nerve can trigger the parasympathetic response to calm the person down and lower the heart rate and blood pressure to bring the body back to a state of normal.

If the anxiety is not severe, it can usually be treated naturally by incorporating various relaxation techniques into a daily routine. But severe anxiety should be treated medically and may be done so with a device that sends electrical pulses directly to the vagus nerve.

- Addiction

Researchers at the University of Texas, Dallas, School of Behavioral and Brain Sciences, studied breaking the behavioral cycles of addition with vagus nerve stimulation. This research, which began in 2017, found that vagus nerve stimulation supported the 'extinction learning' behavioral pattern of drug-seekers. Stimulating the vagus nerve reduced the cravings better than weaning the user off drugs by slowly reducing their cocaine intake.

Vagus nerve stimulation that was tested on cocaine-addicted lab rats saw a change in the synaptic plasticity connecting the amygdala and the prefrontal cortex. The vagus nerve is stimulated directly by a mild electric current produced by a medical device, approved by the FDA, that gets surgically implanted beneath the skin.

- Alzheimer's

The stimulation of the vagus nerve can restore cognitive function. A study that ran from June 2000 to September 2003 showed that after 1 year of vagus nerve stimulation, most of the 17 patients undergoing the test reported at least no decline from their baseline. While some of the patients showed improvement.

The treatment itself showed that the patients tolerated vagus nerve stimulation well, with no decline or upsets in the patient's quality of life.

- Autism

Most patients who have neurodevelopmental disorders have been found to have a low vagal tone. Further studies showed that increasing vagal tone by using Vagus Nerve Stimulation (VNS) can give quite significant improvements in the patient's quality of life after therapy. Along with developmental therapies, VNS could potentially allow the patient to be able to communicate, socialize, and study a lot better.

- Chronic Fatigue and Fibromyalgia

Because the vagus nerve regulates many systems in the body, the immune system being one of them, it may be helpful in treating both chronic fatigue syndrome and fibromyalgia.

Vagus nerve stimulation plays a big part in getting rid of pain and is why regular stimulation is useful in helping with the management of fibromyalgia. There are certain areas of the vagus nerve that are responsible for reducing 'temporal summation' which is a process that plays a big part in 'chronic pain states'.

Think of temporal summation as a lasso, parts of the nervous system responsible for pain are lassoed together by temporal summation. Then temporal summation gradually tightens the lasso, and with each squeeze, the body becomes more and more sensitive to pain.

Vagus nerve stimulation has been found to help unwind the central nervous system from the tight embrace of temporal summation to gradually desensitize it to pain.

Chronic fatigue is linked to Fibromyalgia, and the two work in hand and hand. Just as vagus nerve stimulation works to alleviate the symptoms of Fibromyalgia, it can do the same for chronic fatigue syndrome.

- Depression disorder

As shown by a study published in 2016, treatment of Major Depressive Disorder (MDD) with vagus nerve stimulation had some positive results. Vagus nerve stimulation improved the connectivity of the Default Mode Network (DMN) in the brain.

- Epilepsy

Patients who have received vagus nerve stimulation have reported an improvement in their quality of life. Vagus nerve stimulation decreases the frequency of the seizures as well as the intensity of the seizures. Patients who underwent the therapy have claimed they feel less sleepy during the day and have better cognitive memory.

Vagus nerve therapy for the control of epilepsy is done by a vagus nerve stimulator device. The device is implanted beneath the skin with a wire that runs to the vagus nerve and is wound around it. The device acts similar to that of a pacemaker for the heart, except the VNS stimulator sends mild electrical energy impulses to the brain at regular intervals.

The device operates in such a way that the patient who has the implanted device is not aware of it. If they feel a seizure coming on all they need to do is use a magnet to swipe over the device. This action will send an extra pulse boost which, in turn, may lessen the intensity of the seizure or prevent it altogether.

• Migraines and Cluster Headaches

While everyone who suffers from migraines may exhibit some basic similar symptoms, for the most part, no two migraines are alike. They can be anywhere from mild blurred vision, nausea, and discomfort to a full-blown raging pain that makes a person feel like their skull is going to explode. What is worse with this kind of migraine is that if it has developed to this stage there is sure to be nausea and vomiting. Vomiting becomes both a relief and a curse as the pain escalates each time a person vomits.

Vagus nerve therapy was applied in a study as a treatment for chronic migraines and acute cluster headache patients. The non-invasive vagus nerve stimulator targeted the back of the head to stimulate the vagus nerve's cervical branch.

It proved to be effective where most of the patients reported a reduction in pain while others reported no pain at all.

- OCD and PTSD

Both OCD and PTSD patients in various trials showed between 40 to 50 % improvement with vagus nerve stimulation. After a year-long trial, patients with OCD, PTSD, and Personality Disorder (PD) showed continued improvement with regular treatment and an implanted device.

- Rheumatoid arthritis

A study that was conducted in 2016, by experts of immunology in conjunction with neuroscientists on Vagus Nerve Stimulation (VNS), found that the treatment blocked the production of pro-inflammatory cytokines. When pro-inflammatory cytokines cannot be produced it reduces the inflammatory reflex.

This reduces inflammation and cytokines in rheumatoid arthritis patients.

- Traumatic brain injury

Traumatic brain injury (TBI) is when some form of injury to the brain causes the neurons to disconnect and then atrophy. Traumatic brain injury has a high mortality rate, especially in military personnel.

There are not many treatments for traumatic brain injury, and depending on the severity, it can leave a person with limited conscious state or in a vegetative state. Upon approval from the FDA to implant vagus nerve stimulators in patients with traumatic brain injury, a study was conducted examining the use of this in TBI patients. This study showed that the stimulation of the vagus nerves affects the stimulation of blood flow to various parts of the brain in order to improve consciousness.

PUTTING IT ALL TOGETHER

We mentioned in about how all of the systems work together in harmony to create all of the body processes that living organisms need to survive. We will launch further into this and discuss how the vagus nerve can actually modulate different body systems through its functionality and parasympathetic effects. We will break this chapter down into specific systems and discuss how the vagus nerve works with and benefits that particular organ system. The vagus nerve supplies a vast number of benefits for the human body, and we will get more in-depth in that here.

Since the nerve innervates many different sections and organs of the body, it will directly impact multiple organ systems. Furthermore, since the vagus nerve is the main component of the parasympathetic nervous system, it effectively impacts every area of the body either directly or indirectly. A living organism is one big cycle of reciprocity where all of the body systems give and receive as needed to maintain their own functionality. The vagus nerve works in conjunction with many of the body systems, and that is what we will discuss today. Here are some of them.

The Endocrine System

The endocrine system in the body produces chemical substances called hormones that regulate the activity of certain cells and organs of the body. These activities include growth, metabolism, and sexual development and function. This is done by sending chemical messages between different cells to control particular physiological processes. The endocrine system is made up of multiple glands that secrete hormones into the bloodstream. These hormones move throughout the body, controlling certain emotions and behaviors. When one hormone from a particular gland arrives at the receptor of another gland, it triggers the gland to release other hormones, creating a chain of chemical reactions throughout the body.

Both the sympathetic and parasympathetic nervous systems interact with the endocrine system to elicit chemicals that provide another system for influencing our feelings and behaviors. The endocrine system plays a vital role in controlling our emotions. The various hormones released through the different glands incite many different responses by the body. In essence, the endocrine system may control the parasympathetic nervous system in this manner. As the endocrine system creates certain hormones, this will cause the parasympathetic response, operated by the vagus nerve, to slow down certain body processes and bring our physiology into a state of calmness. In turn, the parasympathetic nervous system can actually modulate the endocrine response. When the body is in a state of panic and stress created by a sense of danger, certain hormones are released to activate the sympathetic nervous system. During moments of danger, the sympathetic nervous system is working in conjunction with the various endocrine glands to help the body be in a heightened response out od necessity.

Over time, when the sympathetic response is no longer needed, then the parasympathetic response kicks in. The vagus nerve can effectively modulate the endocrine system by counteracting the effects of the sympathetic nervous system, which will reduce the hormone activity that elicited the fight-or-flight response. Here is an example: the body is in a state of panic due to perceived danger. A rise in heart rate, blood pressure, and breathing is needed to overcome a possibly dangerous situation. For example, running away from a threat, which would be the flight response. At this time, the endocrine system has produced and released countless hormones that are needed for the heightened response. When the perceived danger is over, activating the vagus nerve can elicit the parasympathetic response, which will help to shut down the chemical reactions currently occurring and cause the endocrine system to release a different set of hormones. Those are needed to help calm the body down.

Let's take this a step further. We spoke earlier about how certain stimulation exercises can activate the vagus nerve. Being able to do so during a state of panic and stress will effectively alter the course of the endocrine system, changing its current physiological state. We'll explain this a little bit further. While in the middle of a situation that activated our sympathetic response, we begin to do deep breathing exercises. These deep breaths then stimulate the vagus nerve, causing the parasympathetic response to kick in. This parasympathetic response will inhibit the sympathetic response, reducing the heart rate, blood pressure, and breathing. Also, it will speed up digestion. This will also inhibit the endocrine hormones that had been released during the fight-or-flight response, in turn, causing the parasympathetic system to effectively modulate and control the endocrine system.

The endocrine system and the nervous system work very closely together to control many behavioral processes. They work together and can inhibit one another through their own functional practices. The main area we wanted to focus on here is to argue how the vagus nerve could effectively modulate something like the endocrine system. It can do so by activating the parasympathetic response, successfully altering many body processes that control mood and emotions. If it can do this, perhaps it is further proof that the vagus nerve can control mood disorders. We will get more into this later.

The Skeletal System

The skeletal system consists of the bones, tendons, and ligaments of the human body. Its function is to support the body, facilitate movement, protect the internal organs, and produce certain cells. The skeletal system is built and rebuilt constantly throughout our lives during the growth process. Cells known as osteoblasts work to build up the bone density, whereas osteoclasts break down the bone. Both cell types work together to create a structured skeletal system that is capable of performing the functions it needs to. We may take our bones for granted, thinking they are there. However, multiple body processes are occurring to help keep them alive and well.

The question is, how does the vagus nerve fit into all of this. Very strongly, indeed. Since the vagus nerve innervates multiple organs, it is largely responsible for the skeletal muscle to receive the nutrients it needs to function properly. Bone growth is often dependent on movement. With more movement, more bone growth occurs. The vagus nerve may help to inhibit certain body functions, effectively reducing movement and also reducing excessive bone growth.

Finally, the vagus nerve, indirectly, can control the movement of the skeletal system, effectively slowing down the body during times of stress and allowing a recovery and relaxation phase to occur. After the vagus nerve is stimulated and inhibits certain body processes through the activity of the parasympathetic nervous system, it can slow down the body, and slow down the skeletal system, allowing the body to be at rest after a moment of heightened activity. Excessive movement can be good for the skeletal system, as it allows for movement of the joints and other structures. Excessive movement can also become a problem for the breakdown of cartilage and injury to the skeletal bone. The vagus nerve, in its own way, helps to protect the skeletal system by modulating it through the activities of the parasympathetic nervous system.

The Microbiota-Intestinal-Nervous System Axis

The Microbiota-Intestinal-Nervous system axis, more simply know as the Gut-Brain axis, consists of the bidirectional communication between the central and enteric nervous system of the gastrointestinal tract. This links the emotional and cognitive centers of the brains with peripheral intestinal functions. Further research suggests that microorganisms of the gut can affect both the enteric and central nervous systems, which indicates the existence of the microbiota-gut-brain axis. Due to this close relationship of the gut and the brain, many microorganisms found in the gut have been associated with common disorders of the central nervous system, like Parkinson's Disease, Alzheimer's, schizophrenia, and multiple sclerosis.

The microbiota-gut-brain axis also refers to the biochemical communication between the digestive tract and the brain itself. You may have heard the term "gut instinct." Well, there is definitely some validity to this. If your gut and brain are connected in such a way, it suggests that your gut instincts, whether towards people, places, or a situation, are certainly something to take seriously. If something does not feel right, it may not be. Listen to your gut.

How does the vagus nerve fit into all of this? As we mentioned several times before, the vagus nerve is the main component of the parasympathetic nervous system. It is also composed of both afferent and efferent fibers; however, it is heavily skewed towards the afferent fibers, which send information from the peripheries back to the brain. These fibers make up about 80 percent of the vagus nerve, with the rest consisting of efferent fibers. The vagus nerve also innervates much of the intestinal tract, where it ends, while originating in the brain stem. This is the one cranial nerve that literally travels this distance and directly connects the brain to the gut. The vagus nerve also has strong interoceptive awareness or the awareness to sense internal body sensations, which involve the process of receiving, accessing and evaluating internal body signals. For all of these reasons, the vagus nerve is able to sense the metabolic substances in the gut and send the information it receives from them directly up through the afferent fibers back to the brain, instantly creating direct communication between the two systems. We could probably make all sorts of jokes about how the stomach and head are connected, but we will just move along.

What does all of this mean? The vagus nerve is at the interface of the gut-brain axis. The vagus nerve will directly communicate abnormality in the digestive tract to the brain, and the brain will then send down signals through the vagus nerve down to the gut. When communication is not well connected, researchers feel this is when significant diseases may occur. For example, in diseases like irritable bowel syndrome or inflammatory bowel disease, decreased vagal tone was noted. If we work on stimulating the vagus nerve through this axis, we can essentially help to overcome many digestive tract illnesses.

On the flip side, with this strong gut-brain communication, we can also help promote positive mood by understanding and supporting our health in the gastrointestinal tract. Abnormal microbiota in the gut has been one of the biggest links to depressive disorders, and many researchers feel that correcting this dysfunction can lead to significant inhibition of depression. Due to this, a large focus has been placed on the brain-gut axis for helping to alleviate mood disorders like depression.

How Does This All Link?

Since further research is continuing to show that depression is not simply a problem in the brain, more of an emphasis is being placed on improving the health of other systems. This will effectively help with depression. This connection strongly indicates a physical component to depression, rather than just a mental one. The immune system, endocrine system, nervous system, and digestive system all play a role in depression. The brain-gut access, controlled strongly by the vagus nerve, provides a strong indication between the links of physical disorders and mental disorders.

One of the things that all of the systems mentioned above have in common is that they are all linked in some way to the wandering vagus nerve. If we have not been able to drive home the importance of the vagus nerve up to this point, we hope to do it right here, right now. Since the vagus nerve starts in the brain stem and ends in the digestive tract, we already know that it strongly links the two systems directly. Therefore, any dysfunction in the gut can be directly communicated to, and effect, the central nervous system. Many of the disorders of the two systems have been associated with a weak vagal tone, further suggesting that stimulating the vagus nerve will directly impact and improve the dysfunction of the brain and gut. This will effectively help to reduce depression as well.

Furthermore, the vagus nerve plays a huge role in the inflammatory process associated with the immune system. Excessive and uncontrolled inflammation has been strongly linked to depression and mood disorders. The increased vagal tone has been linked to a decrease in inflammation. In conclusion, stimulating the vagus nerve properly will help to inhibit inflammation, effectively improving depression. With poor diets and often sedentary lifestyles, inflammation is becoming a greater cause for concern. If we can simply inhibit inflammation by stimulating the vagus nerve naturally, it can do wonders for our physical and mental health. This further shows just how much the nerve can improve our lives in a variety of ways.

Finally, let's talk about the endocrine system. We mentioned how the endocrine system functions through various glands, sending countless hormones throughout the body. Certain hormones that are released during the sympathetic response can create a stressful situation, and when the body is under constant stress, depression, and mood disorders will occur. In order to counteract the sympathetic response, we must stimulate the parasympathetic response through activation of the vagus nerve. This response will inhibit the sympathetic nervous system and also reduce the stress-causing hormones produced by the endocrine system. Hormones are truly produced by the body based on the most critical functions at the time. Stimulating the vagus nerve will help to relax the body and produce the proper hormones to help inhibit the physiological processes.

Calming down the body through stimulation of the vagus nerve can also loosen up the musculoskeletal tract. This will further help to reduce stress, pain, and mood disorders. The various systems work together via the functions of the vagus nerve to help reduce the heightened responses of the body. Effectively utilizing the vagus nerve can help to improve many body processes

The parasympathetic and sympathetic nervous systems work together to create a homeostasis in the body. Meaning, they balance out the physiological processes and responses based on the situation that is occurring. Just like with a bike, sometimes you need to peddle, sometimes you need to break. Sometimes the body needs to stimulate the sympathetic nervous system; sometimes, it needs to stimulate the parasympathetic nervous system. In reality, both are working all of the time; it is just that one will overtake the other in times of need. The parasympathetic nervous system inhibits and slows down functions throughout the entire body. Since the vagus nerve is the main element of the parasympathetic nervous system, it also helps to control most of the body. The vagus nerve is truly a giant, both physically and functionally. To ignore its significance is to ignore our health and well-being.

Can A Breath Make You Better?

There is one last section we want to cover here, and that is the idea of breathing and mood. We spoke extensively about the benefits of conscious breathing and the vagus nerve. We want to further drive home the point here about how taking simple breaths can improve our functionality in so many ways. It can help put us in a calmer state and also improve our ability to communicate. Remember that taking a deep breath stimulates the vagus nerve, causing the parasympathetic nervous system to kick in. The parasympathetic nervous system will inhibit and lower the heart rate, blood pressure, and breathing. It will also relax the smooth muscle in the body. Overall, this will put our bodies in a calmer state. When our bodies are in a calmer state, we are able to think more clearly. When we are able to think more clearly, we can express our thoughts better, and this will help to improve our communication.

When we are in distress or panic, so many things are happening inside of us so quickly. We are in a state of heightened response, which is needed when we quickly have to escape danger. However, when we need to get our thought together, we need to slow everything down. We do this by stimulating the vagus nerve. That being said, the question is, can a minute or less of deep breathing put us in a calmer state and help us communicate better? The answer is yes. Even just a few deep breaths will begin to stimulate the vagus nerve, which in turn will begin to inhibit the sympathetic response. This instant change will allow us to begin thinking more clearly and communicating properly. The answer then is a resounding, yes! A minute or even just a few seconds of deep breathing can put our bodies in a calmer state and improve our communication skills. Of course, a speech class would be helpful, as well.

Let's look at a scenario real quick. We have probably seen this in almost every action movie. A person is in grave danger and needs to get out of a severely dangerous situation. He runs, jumps, climbs, or fights and does whatever he needs to do to get out of the dangerous situation. During this time, his sympathetic nervous system is in full mode as he is in the fight-or-flight response. As soon as he is able to find a safe place to hide, he begins taking deep breaths to calm himself and his body down. By doing this, he can collect his thoughts and decide the next course of action. At this moment, his parasympathetic nervous system has kicked in.

As we can see, both systems are equally valuable and necessary to sustain life. If one is dysfunctional, the body will become dysfunctional. The key is to keep the body in a state of balance where the two systems are counteracting each other. We spoke earlier about how we can suppress the sympathetic response by stimulating the vagus nerve. In reality, this is probably not a good idea when you need the sympathetic nervous system to get you out of a dangerous situation. Find the appropriate times to activate the vagus nerve and use it to your advantage. If you did not know about the vagus nerve before, we hope that you do now. If you are not feeling right, perhaps you need to sit down and take a deep breath.

CONCLUSION

As we have seen in this last list, there is one aspect that should undoubtedly call our attention: the simple fact of cultivating positive emotions, such as enjoying good social relationships, having moments of leisure, laughter and relaxation, It also offers a very beneficial stimulus in our vagus nerve.

We cannot forget that it is in the intestine itself that between 80 and 90% of serotonin, the well-being hormone, is manufactured. Nor can we ignore that the mere fact of drawing a smile on the face, dancing, walking, swimming, etc., generates very positive metabolic changes. Changes that this immense nerve, which "wanders" erratically through our body, instantly captures to send a very concrete message to our brain: "Everything is calm, we are fine."

You do not need to be controlled by your body and mind. Because you have the power to tell them what to do

By stimulating your vagus nerve yourself, you can send a message to your body telling it's time to relax. In the long term, this will improve your mood and increase your resilience, resilience and well-being.

The increase in the tone of my vagus nerve has allowed me and overcome my depression and also to deal with symptoms better if they were to occur again.

ιformation can be obtained
˜Gtesting.com
˙he USA
˙38030321
˙00003B/562

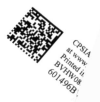

CPSIA
at www.
Printed ii
BVHW08
601496B